kettlebell exercises that make kettlebells such a versatile and effective tool to train with.

This guide not only covers the kettlebell swing but also other important beginners information like what kettlebell to get etc. this makes it the perfect guide to read for a beginner and have all the important information needed in one place.

Comes with many detailed step-by-step photos and diagrams.

Answers to questions like:

How to swing a kettlebell without injuring myself?
How to workout with kettlebell swings?
How many swings should I do?
What muscles are worked with the kettlebell swing?
What kettlebell weight should I start with?
What kettlebell to choose?
How do I warm-up for kettlebell swings?

+7 AWESOME
KETTLEBELL SWING WORKOUTS

Table of Contents

Important 6

About the Author 7

Step 1: Perfect the Bodyweight Hip Hinge 10

    The Ankles Remain in a Neutral Position and Do Not Bend 12

    The Shins Remain Vertical 14

    The Knees Bent to Bring the Hips Back 15

    The Hips Bent to Bring the Shoulders Down 16

    The Back Remains Neutral 17

    The Neck Remain Neutral 18

    The Shoulders Are Slightly Pulled Back 19

    The Arms Hang 20

Step 2: Perfect the Hip Hinge Deadlift 22

    The Weight Is Placed Right Under the Arms 24

    The Grips on the Handle Are Loose 25

    The Arms Just Hang and Do Not Lift the Weight 26

    The Spine Is Kept Straight with a Rigid Structure Around It 27

    The Pelvis Is the Structure That You Want to Move to Lift 28

    The Muscles Around the Buttocks Do the Main Lifting 29

    The Hamstrings and Adductor Magnus Are Another Group That Powers the Lift 29

    A Neutral Standing Position Is Feet Under the Shoulders 33

Step 3: Perfect the Kettlebell Swing 34

    Place the Weight at the Correct Distance 36

    Delay the Hip Hinge 37

    The Kettlebell Remains an Extension of the Arms 38

    The Top Part of the Swing Can Be Compared to a Plank Position 39

    Kettlebell Swing Step-By-Step in Pictures 40

Step 4: Increasing Reps/Weight 44

    Endurance 44

    Power 45

    Strength 45

    Volume 45

Step 5: Working out with Kettlebell Swings 47

Step 6: Time to Venture Further 58

    Bonus 61

THE QUICK AND CONCISE KETTLEBELL SWING GUIDE

The kettlebell swing, burn fat and build muscle at the same time.

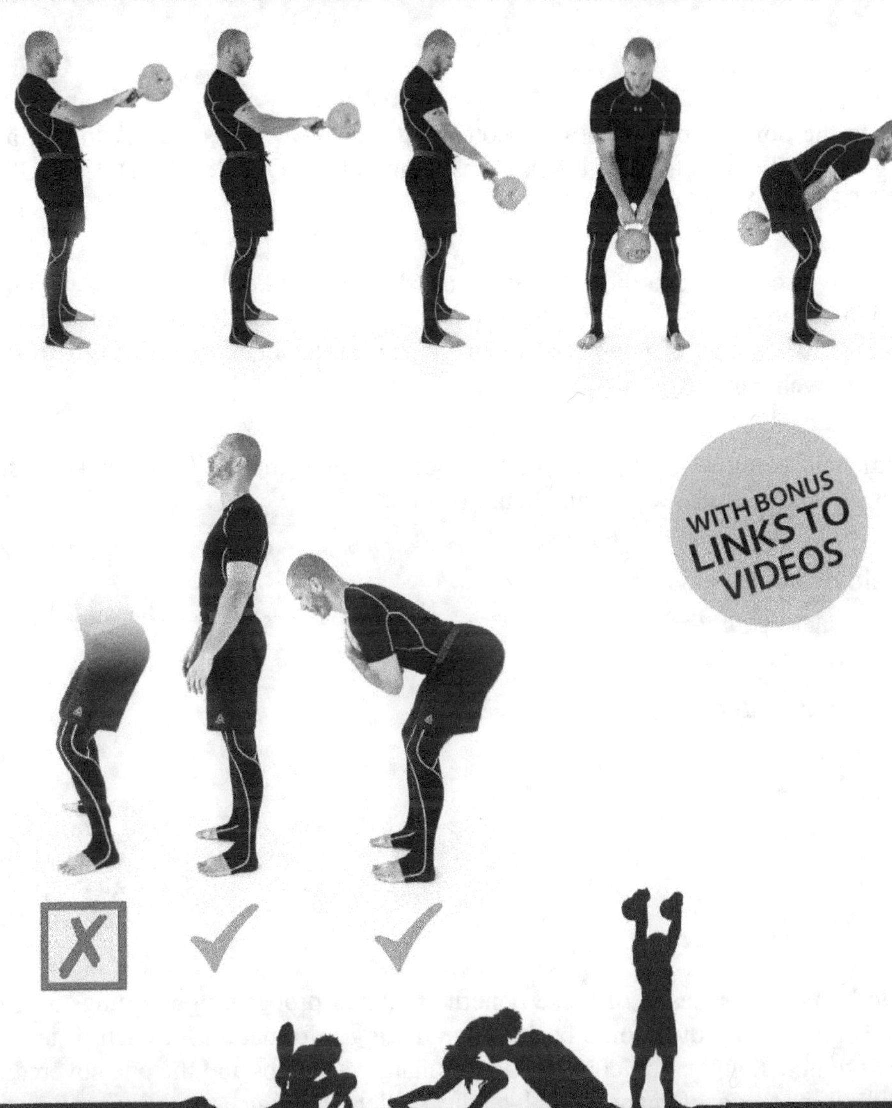

By Taco Fleur from Cavemantraining

The Quick And Concise Kettlebell Swing Guide

The kettlebell swing, burn fat and build muscle at the same time.

Straight to the point information and photos that will have you safely swinging and working out with a kettlebell quicker than any other QUICK AND CONCISE KETTLEBELL SWING GUIDE.

This guide will cover the popular conventional double-arm kettlebell swing which is the version of the kettlebell swing where you hold on to the kettlebell with two hands and perform a hip hinge movement to move the kettlebell back and forth in one explosive movement.

The kettlebell swing is by far one of the most popular and well-known kettlebell exercises. It's an exercise with many benefits, like:

- cardiovascular endurance
- muscular endurance
- flexibility
- full body workout
- core strength
- grip strength
- low-impact
- power
- etcetera

It should be noted that each of these benefits requires proper programming to meet goals, this guide will cover some basic programming information for each. It is also important to note that the kettlebell swing has many variations and the one covered in this guide is just one of many, just like the kettlebell swing is only one of many

Personalized Online Coaching 62
What Muscles Are Worked with the Kettlebell Swing?...........................63
    Grip..63
    Posture/shoulders...63
    Spine 63
    Prime movers..64
    Flexion and stabilization...64
Ever Wondered What Exactly Happens During a Kettlebell Swing? 66
    From backswing to up phase 66
    From floating phase to backswing..67
Caveman Kettlebell Swing Muscle Priming Routine...............................68
    Warm-up..68
    Warning 71
    Muscle priming...72
Kettlebell Books 77
    21-Days to Kettlebell Training for Beginners 78
    Kettlebell Workouts and Challenges 1.0 79
    Kettlebell Workouts and Challenges 2.0 80
    Kettlebell Exercise Encyclopedia 81
Become Certified...82
   82
Kettlebell Features And Which Kettlebell To Get? What Size And Weight?........83

Important

Fully master the technique at each step presented in this book before performing higher and/or heavier unbroken repetitions of the kettlebell swing. The steps have been carefully planned and designed after years of teaching thousands of people across the world online and in-person.

To perform a kettlebell swing properly you need to understand not only the movement but also what muscles power and make the movement possible so that you can activate or contract them and keep the exercise safe. This guide will slowly feed all this information to you about the muscles in such a way that it builds up step-by-step to avoid information overload.

Each of the points noted at a step of the progression transfers to the next step in the progression to swinging a kettlebell, remember to transfer the knowledge along to the next step.

In this guide you'll find some external links which start with go.cavemantraining.com, they are short links, i.e. they are used to make long complex links easier to type in. They are case-sensitive though, which means you have to type them in the same case as they appear, in other words, go.cavemantraining.com/ebook is not the same as go.cavemantraining.com/EBOOK.

This collection of information is named *"The Quick And Concise Kettlebell Swing Guide"*. **Quick** as in the information is kept short and to the point to get you started as quickly as possible with the kettlebell swing but in a safe way. **Concise** as in I will be trying to present a lot of information clearly and in a few words; brief but comprehensive. **Guide** as in I will be your guide on this part of your kettlebell journey but also as in a book providing information on a subject.

Whenever the guide calls for the **practice** of a movement/exercise, the amount of reps you will practice remains outside a number that will tax your cardiovascular or muscular endurance. You're training and not working out until you've perfected the technique.

Not only will you be able to rely on the information in this guide but you'll also be able to call upon me for personalized online coaching which can take your kettlebell swing to the next level.

About the Author

My name is Taco Fleur, and I'm a Russian Girevoy Sport Institute Kettlebell Coach, IKFF Certified Kettlebell Trainer, Kettlebell Level 1 + 2 Trainer, Kettlebell Science and Application, HardstyleFit Kettlebell Level 1 Instructor, CrossFit Level 1 Trainer, CrossFit Judges Certificate, CrossFit Programming Certificate, MMA Conditioning Level 1, MMA Fitness Level 1 + 2, Punchfit Trainer and Plyometrics Trainer Certified, with a purple belt in Brazilian Jiu Jitsu. Owner of *Cavemantraining*, author of over 10 kettlebell books, courses, and certifications. Author on *BoxRox* and featured in 4 issues of the *Iron Man* magazine. I have owned and set-up 3 functional kettlebell gyms in Australia and Vietnam, and lived in the Netherlands, Australia, Vietnam and Thailand. I'm currently in the US for 3 months and then back to Europe to decide where we will spend some time running workshops and certifications for a while and then discover a new country.

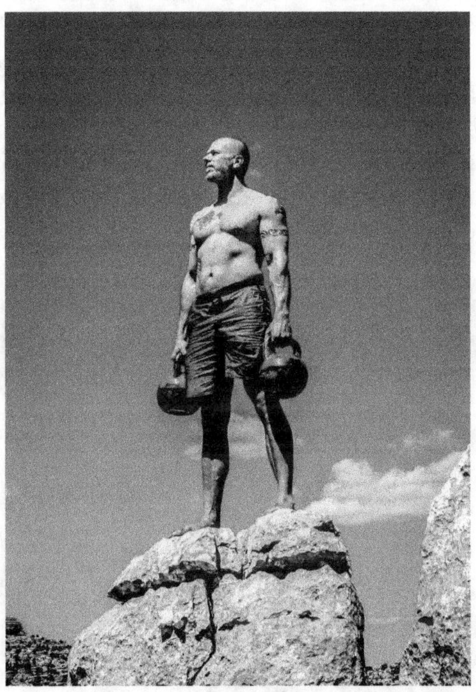

The first thing I'd like you to know about me is that I do **not** know everything, I don't pretend to know everything, and I never will. I'm on a path of life-long learning. I believe there is always something to learn from someone, no matter who they are. I've been physically active since the day I arrived on this earth in 1973. I got serious about training in 1999, touched a kettlebell for the first time in 2004, and got serious about kettlebell training in 2009. I'm here to do what I love most, and that is to share my knowledge with the world.

Some of my personal bests are 400 burpees performed within one hour; 500 kettlebell snatches, 500 swings, and 500 double-unders completed in one session; 250 alternating dead clean and presses in one session with 20kg; 200 pull-ups in one session; 200 unbroken kettlebell swings with a 28kg; most kettlebell swings completed in one session with a 28kg (1,501); most total kettlebell swings done in 28 days with a 28kg (11,111); windmill with a 40kg kettlebell; lugged a kettlebell up a 3,479m mountain; 160kg dead lift; 100 snatches on sand with a 24kg kettlebell; 85kg Olympic Squat Snatch; 300 unbroken clean and jerk with 20kg kettlebell; 10 minute unbroken clean and jerk 79 reps with 2 x 16kg kettlebells; 532 unbroken snatches and achieved rank 2 in kettlebell sport. I mention these PBs not to boast but to demonstrate that I have a good understanding of technique and movement across different areas.

My own training and goals are geared around GPP (General Physical Preparedness) which involves kettlebell training, calisthenics and CrossFit. I like high-volume reps but also like greasing the groove now and again. My main goals are to remains as agile as possible, remaining mobile, training in as many planes of movements as possible, and learning as many different exercise combinations and movements as possible while having fun and enjoying Brazilian Jiu Jitsu. I'm no Arnold Schwarzenegger and never will be, but strength is not solely defined by physical appearance and huge bulging muscles.

You can read more about my training, philosophy, and other ramblings on our website, www.cavemantraining.com, and YouTube channel, bit.ly/youtube-cavemantraining, which as of this writing has over 39,000 subscribers and more than 5 million views.

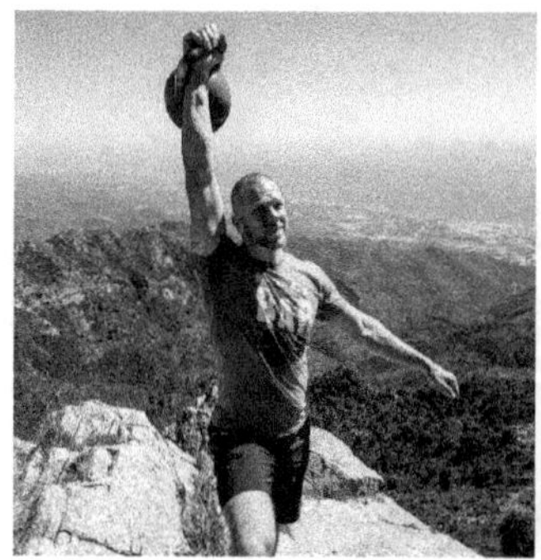
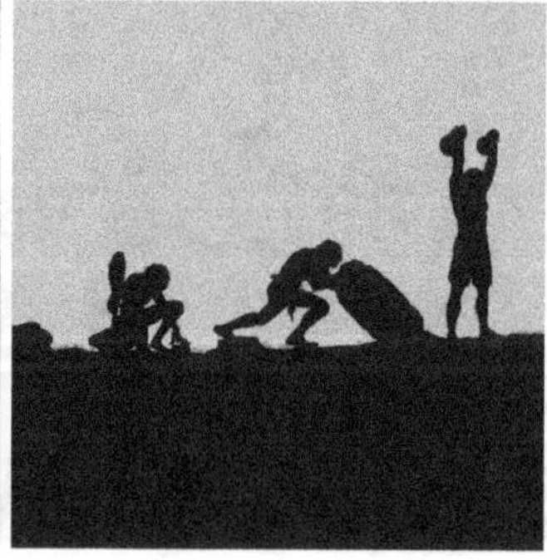
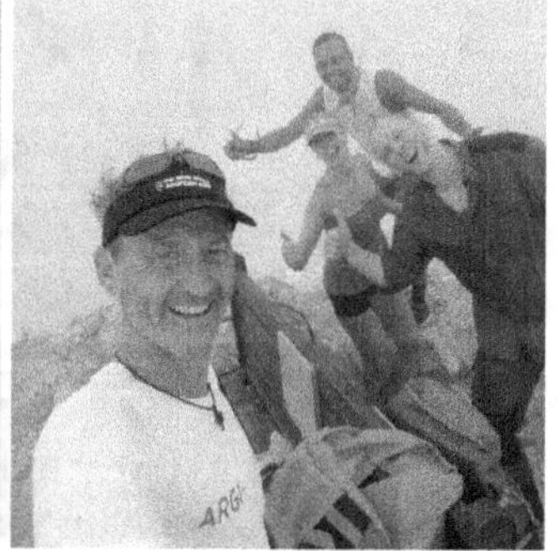

Add me: Facebook.com/taco.fleur or Facebook.com/coach.taco.fleur
Instagram: *@realcavemantraining*

Step 1: Perfect the Bodyweight Hip Hinge

The hip hinge is a movement where the hips, and in our case, the knees come in and out of flexion. See the following photo for an example of the hip hinge.

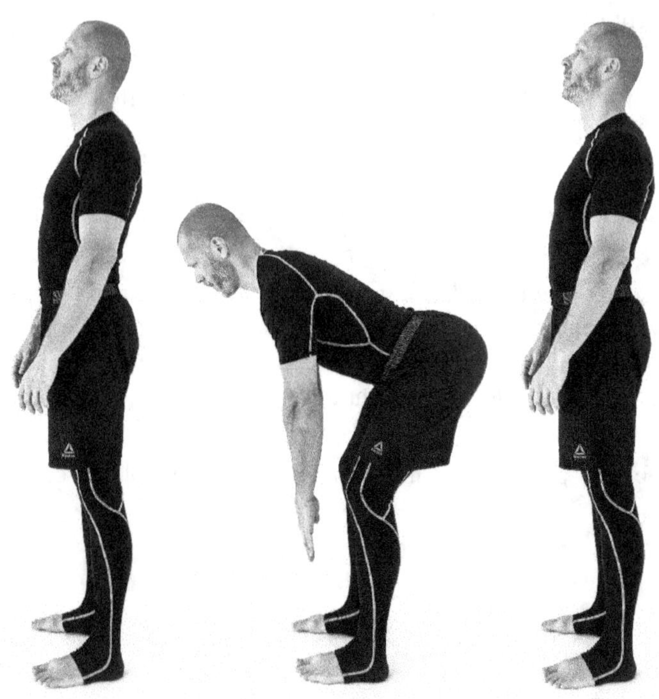

Hip flexion is where the hips fold and extension is the opposite, and the hips are neutral when standing which is always a mixture between flexion and extension. As the hips flex the shoulders move toward the ground and if the hips no longer flex then the shoulders should not move further down.

Practice: Come in and out of the position demonstrated.

A) Neutral standing position

B) Bottom of the hip hinge

C) Neutral standing position

    The Quick And Concise Kettlebell Swing Guide   Taco Fleur

Important points:
- The ankles remain in a neutral position and do not bend
- The shins remain vertical
- The knees bent to bring the hips back
- The hips bent to bring the shoulders down
- The back remains neutral
- The neck remains neutral
- The shoulders are slightly pulled back
- The arms hang

Keep practicing until you understand the movement and have achieved the same or similar position as demonstrated without compromising form. A good way to self assess is by filming yourself side on and then reviewing the movement.

Do not move on to step 2 before perfecting the bodyweight hip hinge.

You are invited to submit your video for assessment in our group here https://go.cavemantraining.com/kettlebells-for-beginners and if you mention this book and tag @Cavemantraining then we will perform the assessment.

What follows are the details of the important dot points listed above.

The Ankles Remain in a Neutral Position and Do Not Bend

The action of the ankles bending is called ankle dorsiflexion, for the hip hinge movement, the ankles should always remain in a neutral position and not bend. In the first photo (left) the ankles are bending and in the second and third photos the ankles remain neutral.

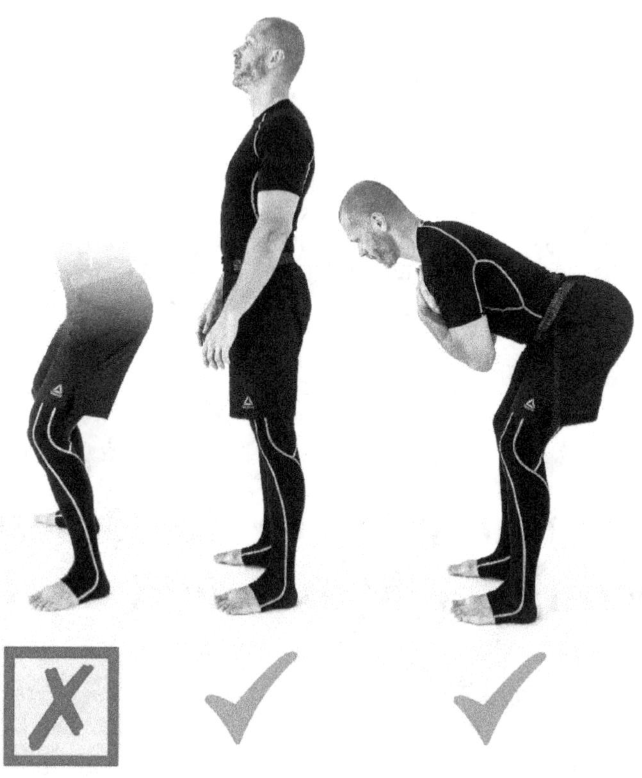

The following demonstrates that the knee joints are no longer positioned above the ankle joints in the first photo (left), whereas in the second photo the knee joints are positioned above the ankle joints, which is correct. None of this means that the knee joints should not bend, it simply means that there should be no movement in the ankle joints during the hip hinge.

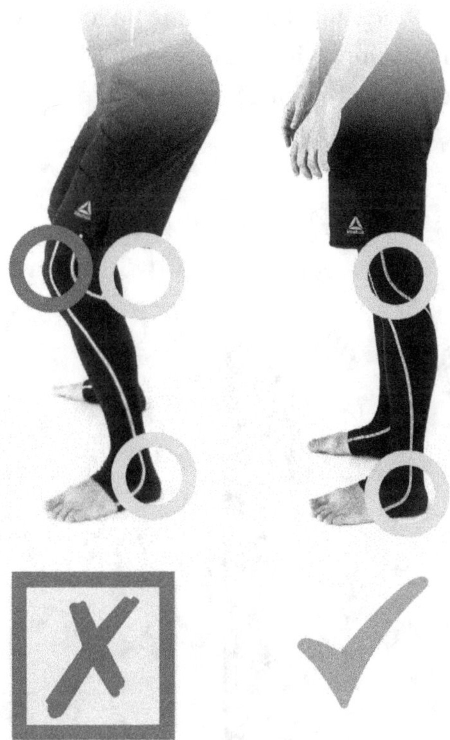

The Shins Remain Vertical

The following photo demonstrates that the shins are no longer vertical but at an angle that is caused by ankle dorsiflexion, which is incorrect. The shins should remain as vertical as possible throughout the hip hinge movement.

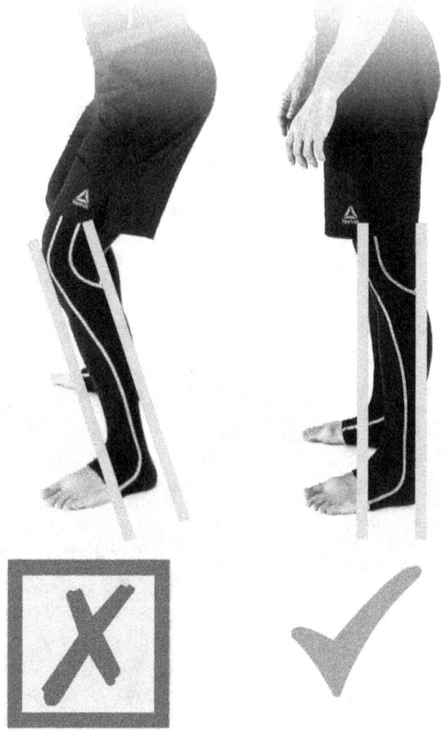

The Knees Bent to Bring the Hips Back

The following photos demonstrate the difference between the hip hinge with straight and bent knees. The first photo (left) demonstrates the hip hinge with straight legs and the second photo (right) with bent knees. The first is also known as a stiff-legged hip hinge or true hip hinge. We will be focussing only on the second version (right).

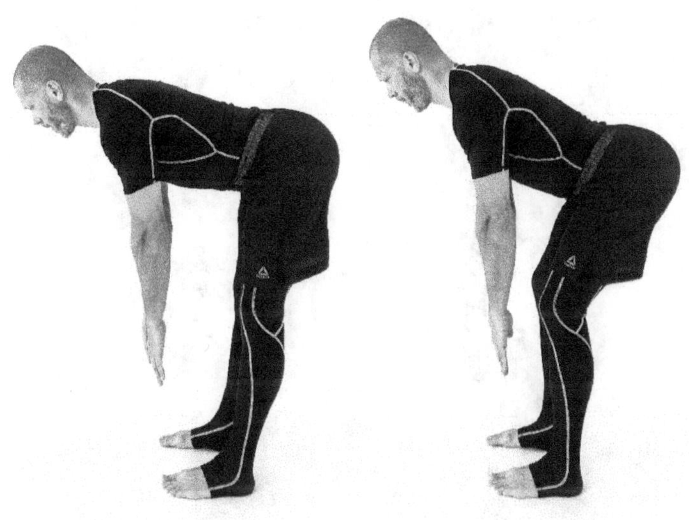

Extended (left) versus flexed (right) knees.

The Hips Bent to Bring the Shoulders Down

The following photo demonstrates how the bending of the hips brings the shoulders closer to the ground. The first photo (left) demonstrates a closer to vertical/upright torso with the sight ahead, which is incorrect for this type of kettlebell swing. The second photo demonstrates a good hip hinge where the torso comes closer to being horizontal. A sight that is ahead (first photo) paired with a close to vertical torso is usually the result of a combination of ankle dorsiflexion and not enough hip flexion.

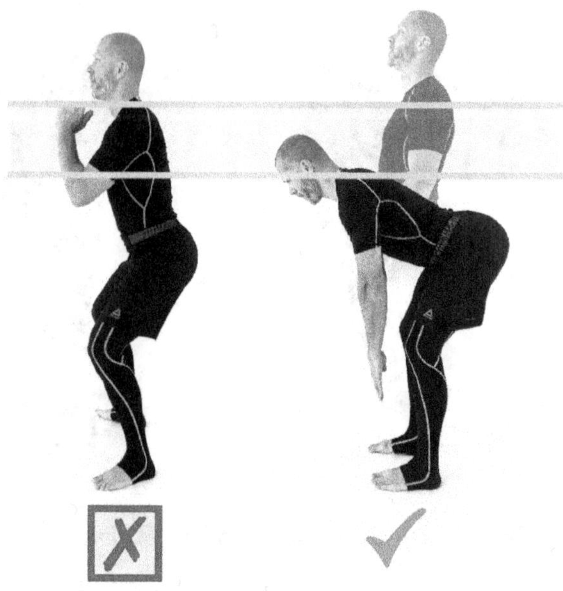

The Back Remains Neutral

The following photo demonstrates how the back/spine remains neutral throughout the movement. If the spine starts to flex during the down phase of the movement then further hip flexion should be aborted. The bending of the spine could be due to tight muscles in the legs or weak muscles in the back, either way, the depth of the hip hinge should only be as deep as proper form allows.

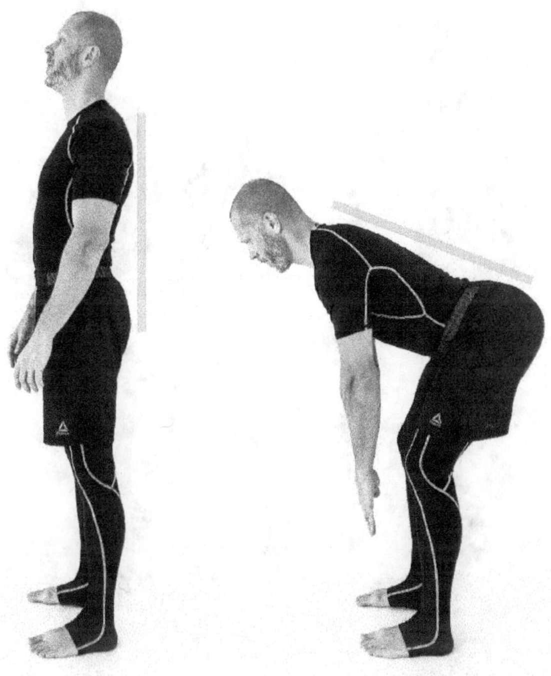

 The Quick And Concise Kettlebell Swing Guide Taco Fleur

The Neck Remain Neutral

The following photo demonstrates how the neck/cervical stays as neutral as possible during the hip hinge. No movement happens in the neck during the hip hinge and the sight changes from straight ahead to down and approx. 1.5m/4feet ahead.

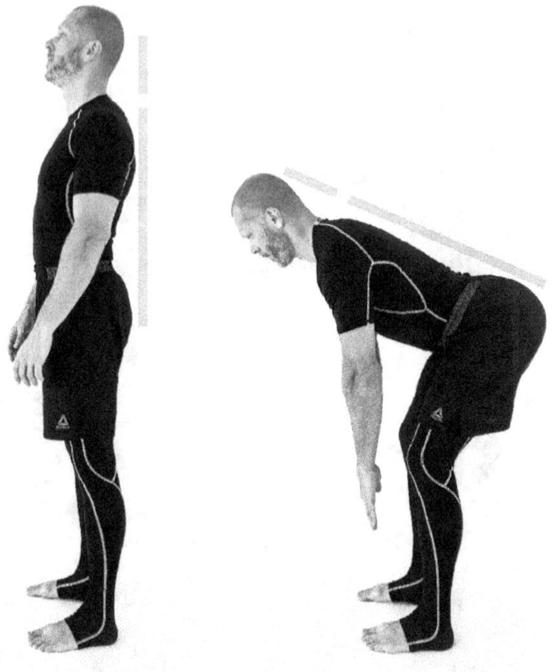

The Quick And Concise Kettlebell Swing Guide

Taco Fleur

The Shoulders Are Slightly Pulled Back

The following photo demonstrates the area that should be working to pull the shoulders slightly back and down. This creates a good structure to eventually hang a weight from.

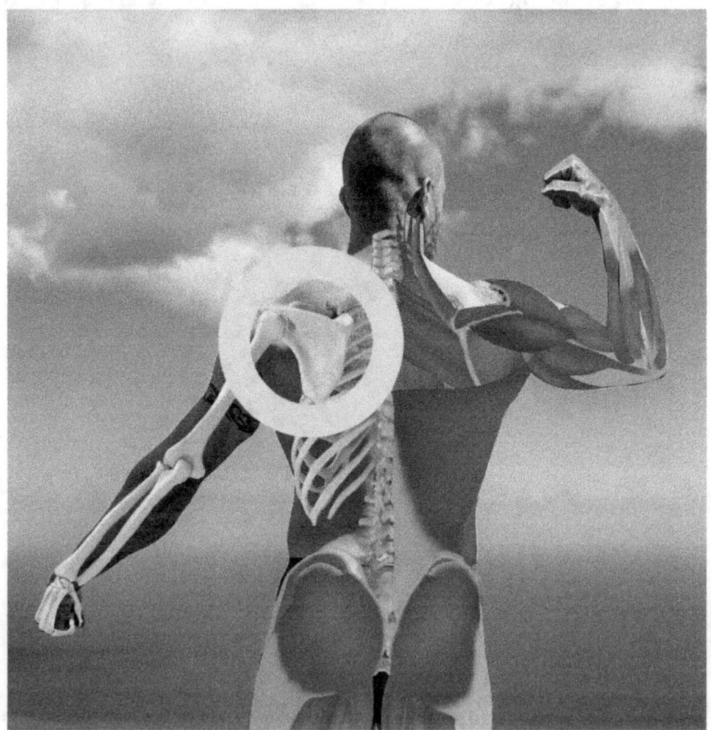

The Arms Hang

The following photo demonstrates how the arms just hang during the hip hinge, you can also bend the elbows and keep the arms in front of your chest, however, it's better to get used to where and how loose the arms should hang for when you start adding weight for the deadlift or swing. Even though the arms should hang relaxed, the slight contraction of the upper back and lats might pull the arms slightly in.

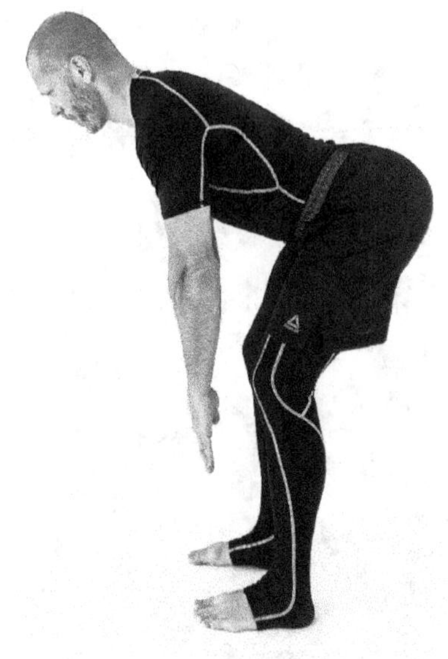

The bodyweight hip hinge viewed at a 45-degree angle.

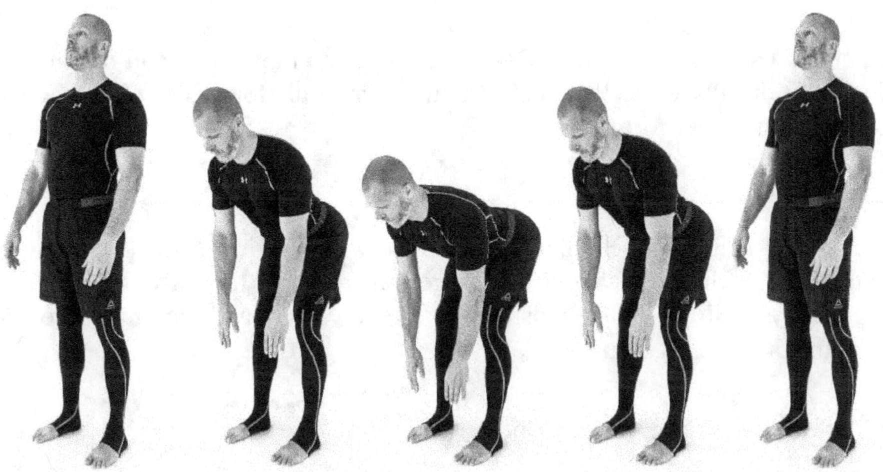

Step 2: Perfect the Hip Hinge Deadlift

Lift a kettlebell dead from the ground with the hip hinge movement and return it to the starting position. Place the kettlebell on an elevated platform if the kettlebell is too low to maintain proper form.

Perform several repetitions of the deadlift exercise with a lightweight. Don't forget that everything from the bodyweight hip hinge transfers and the only difference is that a weight is being lifted which adds load to the movement and requires more and proper recruitment of the right muscles.

Practice: Perform the deadlift as described.

A) Neutral standing position without weight

B) Come into hip flexion

C) Deadlift

D) Neutral standing position with weight

E) Return to dead

F) Neutral standing position without weight

Important points
- The weight is placed right under the arms
- The grips on the handle are loose
- The arms just hang and do not lift the weight
- The spine is kept straight with a rigid structure around it
- The pelvis is the structure that you want to move to perform the lift
- The muscles around the buttocks (located on the posterior of the pelvic region) do the main lifting

- The secondary muscle groups that power the lift are the hamstrings and adductor magnus
- A neutral standing position is feet under the shoulders

Keep practicing until you understand the movement and have achieved approximately 10 consecutive deadlifts without compromising form. A good way to self assess is by filming yourself front and side on and then reviewing the movement.

Do not move on to step 3 before perfecting the bodyweight hip hinge.

You are invited to submit your video for assessment in our group here https://go.cavemantraining.com/kettlebells-for-beginners and if you mention this book and tag @Cavemantraining then we will perform the assessment.

What follows are the details of the important dot points listed above.

The Weight Is Placed Right Under the Arms

The circle in the photo demonstrates approximately where the kettlebell should be placed for deadlifting. The perfect position for the weight is when in the bottom position of the hip hinge there is no need to move the hands to reach for the kettlebell handle.

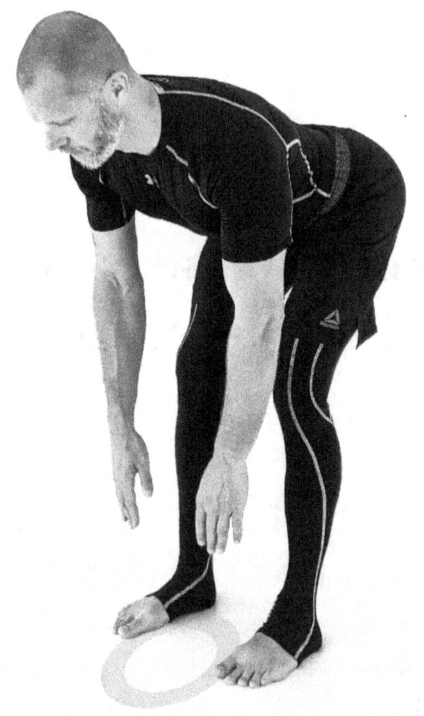

The Grips on the Handle Are Loose

The following photos demonstrate the grips that can be used on the handle. In whatever way the handle is gripped it should be a fairly loose grip and definitely not a tight grip that one would implement for heavyweight farmer walks. The third photo demonstrates a double hand grip with the thumbs placed over the index and middle finger to close the grip and reduce stress on the muscles that flex the fingers (forearms).

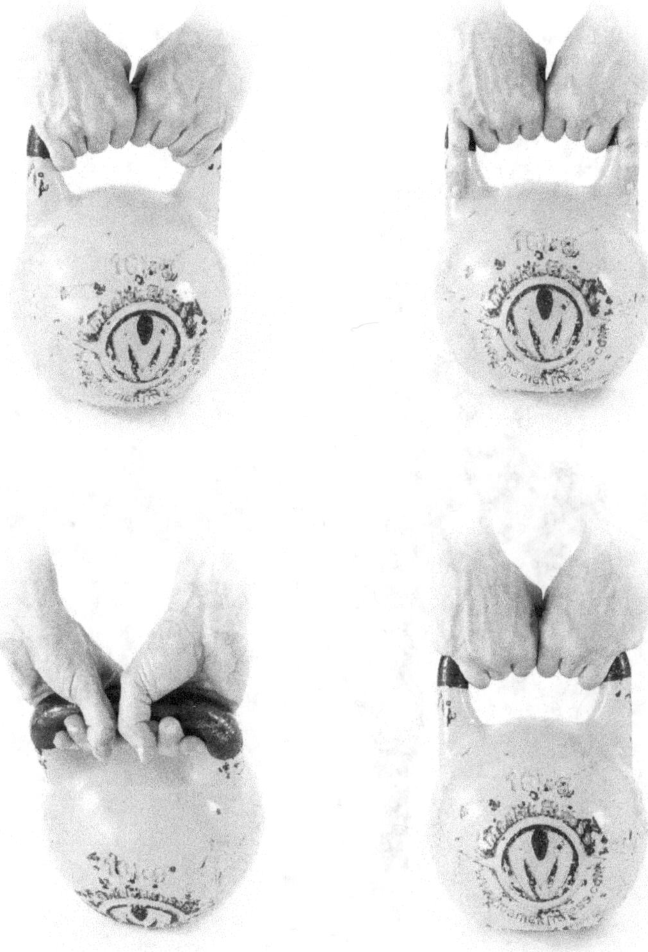

The Arms Just Hang and Do Not Lift the Weight

The lifting of the weight is all done with the muscles at the back from under the lower back down. The elbows should remain straight and should not flex in any way like you're bicep curling the weight. The photo below demonstrates straight arms during a kettlebell swing. It is important to note that as you get more advanced with understanding the kettlebell swing and its variations, it will be possible to swing with a bend in the elbows, for now, the focus is the conventional version of the kettlebell swing.

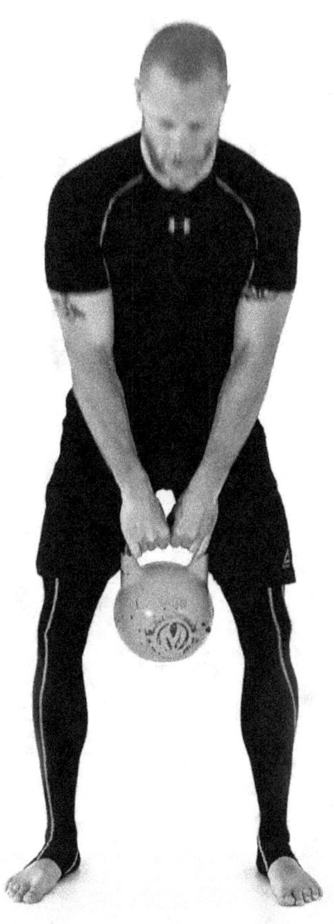

The Spine Is Kept Straight with a Rigid Structure Around It

The muscles that protect the spine, especially the lower back, are super important and require great coverage in this material. The erector spinae are the big muscle groups covering the back and keeping the spine erect, they do their work on the outside but there is also important work that needs to be done on the inside, compression and stabilization around the spine, i.e. creating a solid rigid structure around the spine to keep it from moving.

The spine consists out of 26 bones and is also know as the vertebral column. All these bones and joints allow for movement in many directions, lateral, flexion, extension, rotation, and combinations of those. During the swing any movement in the spine needs to be prevented by the involvement of the right muscles otherwise it means that other muscles can become overloaded and overworked which results in back pain.

Compression needs to be created to protect the spine and prevent movement, this can be thought of as bracing for someone punching you in the abdomen, however, it's important to understand that you're pulling everything in and not pushing it out like you might do when bracing for a blow in the stomach. There are many muscles involved to create the solid structure required during swings, some of them are, but not limited to, transverse abdominal, quadratus lumborum, and internal obliques. The steps to create the structure are:

1. Pull the belly button in
2. Pull the sides in
3. Pull the chest lower to the pelvis

Another way to create that solid structure is by forcing every bit of air out and holding it while breathing behind that solid structure, i.e. retain the structure but keep breathing.

Learn how to create and release the structure at the important points of the movement, for the deadlift that is from lifting to standing neutral, and from standing neutral to returning the weight to dead. At the point the weight is the furthest away from you and the pull starts is when the structure should be the strongest and can relax the further the lift is toward standing neutral. The reverse applies when putting the weight back down, going from relaxed to tighter as the weight reaches the ground. This will also vary depending on how heavy the weight is, in some cases the weight can be so heavy that the spine needs protection throughout the full movement.

The Pelvis Is the Structure That You Want to Move to Lift

For illustration purpose, imagine the bottom of the hip hinge as a closed drawbridge and the hip extensor muscles being the mechanics that pull the drawbridge open, which for our purpose is going from hip extension (closed) to a neutral standing erect position (open).

The bending of the knees is so that the force is not all on the lower back and a type of counterbalance is created, i.e. if the knees remain extended (straight legs) then the shoulders move further away which also brings the weight further away from the closest point possible of being equally balanced. The further the weight is away from that point the more stress there is on the back, especially the lower back, the part of the spine that is just on top of the pelvis (lumbar). Keep these points in mind as they will become extremely important once the movement becomes more explosive, i.e. swinging.

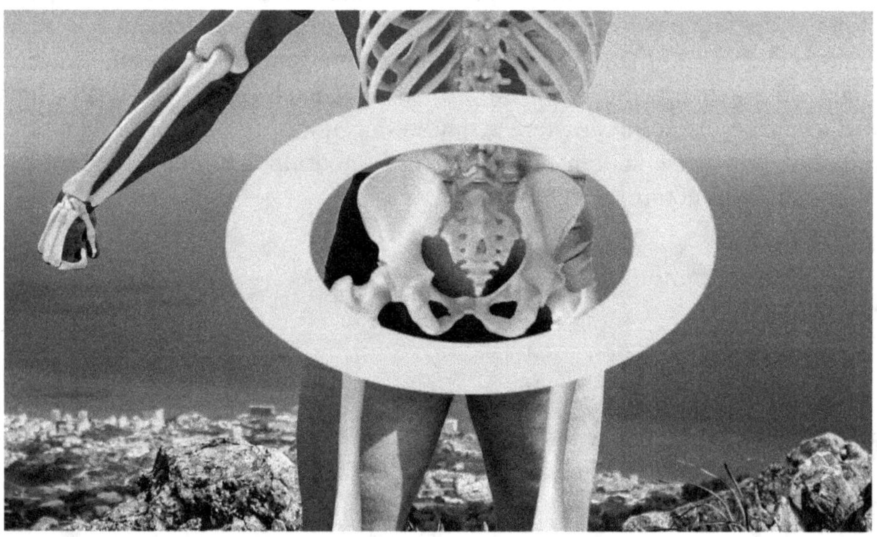

The pelvis.

The pelvis is the structure you want to focus on moving. The hips are the bony structures on each side of the pelvis, each hip bone is comprised of the ilium, ischium, and the pubis.

The Muscles Around the Buttocks Do the Main Lifting

The most important thing about the whole hip hinge movement is knowing what muscles to recruit for actioning the movement, they are the hamstrings, adductor magnus, and gluteus maximus. There are more muscles involved, but these are the prime movers for hip extension. The hamstrings are located at the back of the upper legs. The adductor magni (plural for magnus) are located on the inside thigh areas. The glutei maximi (plural for gluteus maximus) are one of three gluteal muscles in the buttocks and they're connected to the hip bone and the femur (upper leg), contraction of this gluteal muscle powers hip extension, which can also be thought of as pulling the pelvis upright.

The Hamstrings and Adductor Magnus Are Another Group That Powers the Lift

The other muscles like the hamstrings and adductor magni though contraction are responsible for creating a pull at the bottom of the hip bone. Collectively all these muscles and the gluteus maximus can also be referred to as hip extensors, the muscles that extend the hips.

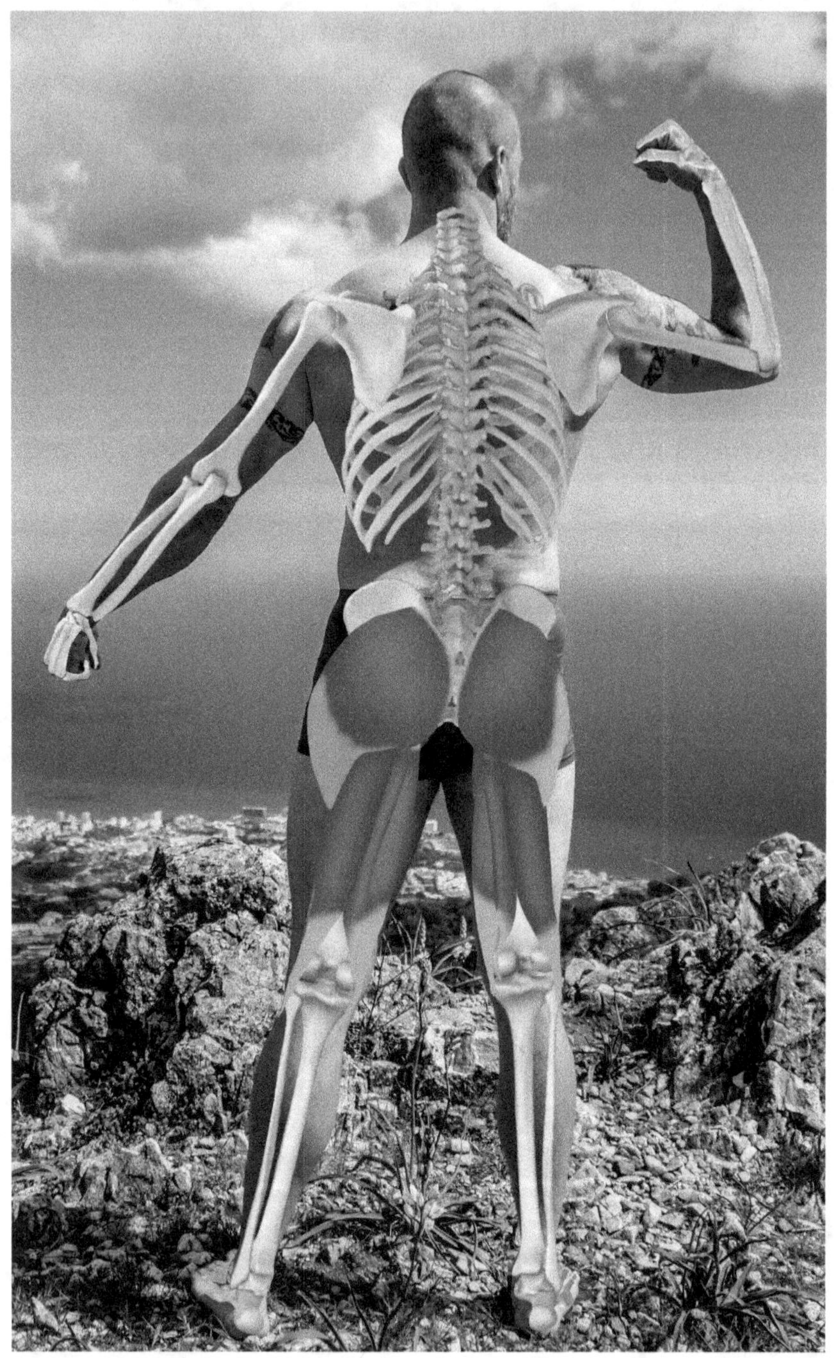

The hip extensor muscles.

Last but not least, the other prime movers involved are for knee extension which is part of the hip hinge used for conventional deadlifts/swings, they are the quadriceps, which is a collection of four muscles on the front of the upper leg (thigh).

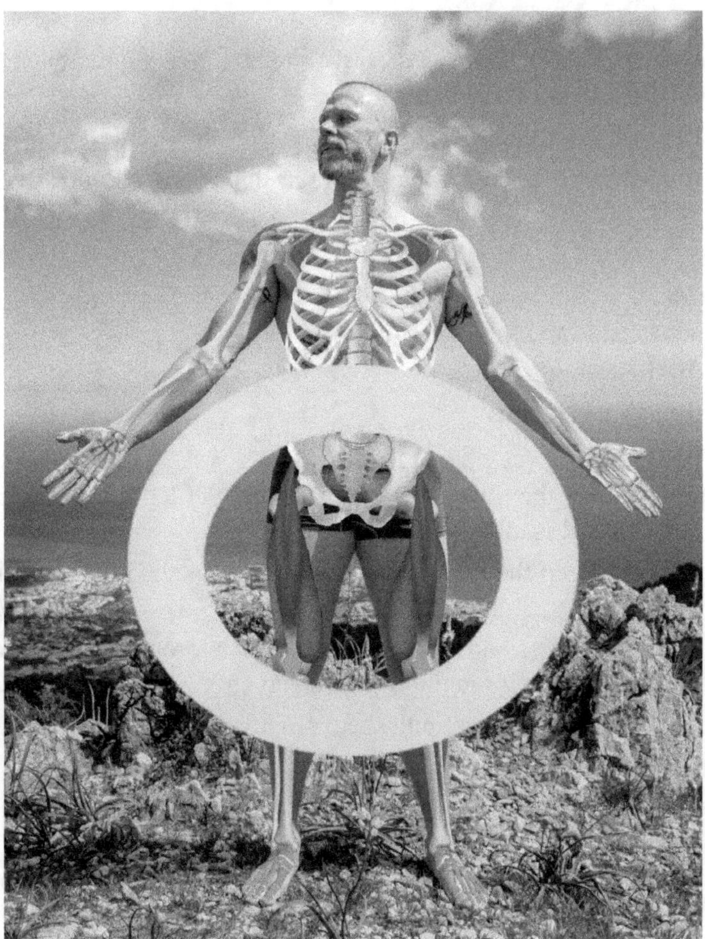

The quadriceps muscle groups.

The muscles that action the movement (prime movers) for the kettlebell swing have been covered but the kettlebell swing is a full-body exercise, meaning that just about every muscle in the body is used at some stage, if not as the prime mover but as a muscle that keeps the body in place so that the intended movement can be created.

Following are some of those muscles that work to stabilize the body while the prime movers do their work to move the kettlebell:

- The calf muscles (back lower leg) keep the shins vertical while the kettlebell is moving at the front
  - Gastrocnemius
  - Soleus
  - Tibialis posterior
  - Flexor digitorum longus
  - Flexor hallucis longus
  - Plantaris
- The muscles along the tibia and fibula (front lower leg) keep the shins vertical while the kettlebell is moving at the back
- The quadriceps keep the hips from falling down as the hips move back (knees flex)
- The transversospinales and erector spinae muscle groups (muscles of the back) keep the spine straight throughout the movement
- Muscles around the scapulae pull them slightly down and together to keep the shoulders safe and back

All these stabilizing muscles contract and release, some stay longer contracted, all contract the most at the highest point of force in the opposing direction.

A Neutral Standing Position Is Feet Under the Shoulders

Although the most common feet position is under the shoulders, it might slightly vary from person to person, in general, try and place the feet under or just slightly outside of the shoulders, meaning, if you would draw a straight line down from your shoulders, the bottom of the line would be in the middle of your feet. Whatever you do, you want to be just wide enough so that the kettlebell can comfortably pass through the legs and not have any part hitting the legs. You want to make sure you are not going wider than you have to either, as this would take away from the power generation and potentially bring along other issues. Your feet will be <u>slightly</u> turned out.

Step 3: Perfect the Kettlebell Swing

The conventional deadlift was used as the natural progression to the kettlebell swing which is the same movement but more explosive, dynamic, and with forces pulling from different directions.

Practice: Perform the kettlebell swing as described.

A) Neutral standing position with the weight placed in front

B) Come into hip flexion

C) Grab hold of the handle

D) Pull the kettlebell back

E) Pull the kettlebell out

F) Stand up straight

G) Propel the kettlebell forward

H) Wait for the kettlebell to fall

I) Wait until the kettlebell is close and then break at the hips and knees

J) Push the kettlebell through the legs

K) Repeat all steps from *E)* onward to keep swinging

L) Reverse step *D)* to *A)* to stop swinging

Important points
- Place the weight at the correct distance
- The arms should connect with the body on the backswing

- Delay the hip hinge
- The kettlebell remains an extension of the arms
- The top part of the swing can be compared to a plank position

Keep practicing until you understand the movement and have achieved 10 consecutive kettlebell swings without compromising form. A good way to self assess is by filming yourself side on and then reviewing the movement.

Place the Weight at the Correct Distance

The weight should be placed at such a distance that there is no need to overreach and compromise form but also far enough to be able to pull it in and back. If the kettlebell is placed near the feet then there is no space between you and the kettlebell for pulling, it will then become an awkward push in.

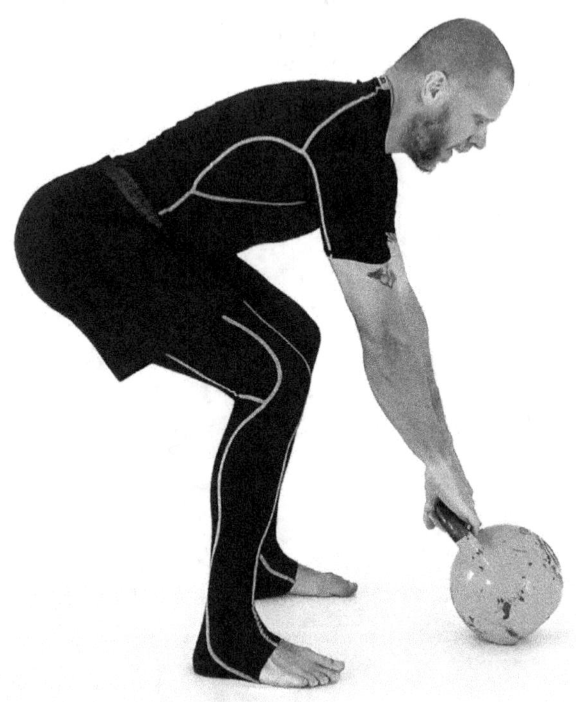

Create some tension between the body and the weight before pulling it back through the legs, slightly lean back to create that tension. Always keep the shoulders higher than the hips. Remember, it's ok to squat for this first rep if it means that is what's required to maintain good form and prevent injury.

  The Quick And Concise Kettlebell Swing Guide Taco Fleur

Delay the Hip Hinge

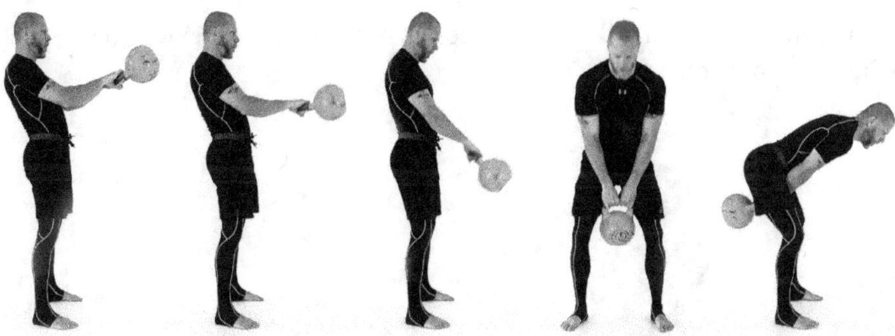

The delay of hip flexion as demonstrated above is the biggest technique point that will help prevent lower back pain and injuries. Remember, as covered earlier, the further the weight is away from the body the more force there is on the posterior. Initiating hip flexion (bending at the hips) as late as possible is what creates a more counterbalanced position and prevents undue stress on the lower back.

1) the top of the swing
2) still in full extension but the kettlebell is falling back down
3) still in full extension with kettlebell nearing the point of breaking at the hips
4) the break at the hips happens
5) the kettlebell is inserted with further hip flexion

The Kettlebell Remains an Extension of the Arms

Control the trajectory of the kettlebell such that it remains an extension of the arms throughout the movement.

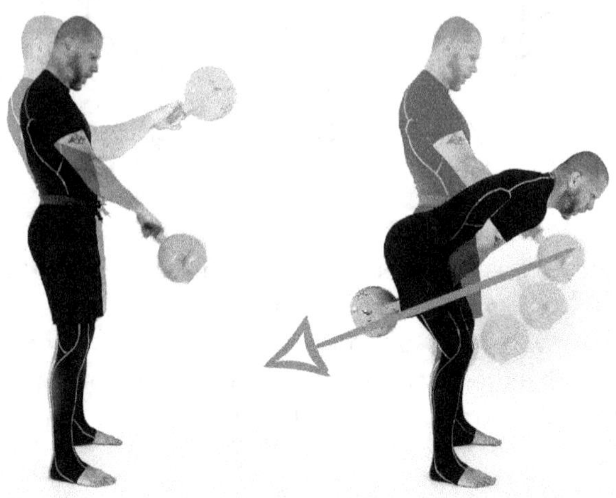

a) Delay hip flexion. b) Create hip flexion and insert the kettlebell.

The arrow represents the direction in which the kettlebell should be pushed, this is important to avoid kettlebell bobbing, which is a quick short movement up and down that the kettlebell would make if the kettlebell is not guided toward the back but instead would finish a half circular pattern. Bobbing of the kettlebell creates friction within the hands and can eventually create excessive callus or blisters.

The Top Part of the Swing Can Be Compared to a Plank Position

If you've been filming yourself and found that you were leaning back or not coming into full extension then the plank is a great way to understand what the top of the swing should be like. The activation of the chest and everything around the scapulae is especially a good example of how the plank position compares to the top of a swing.

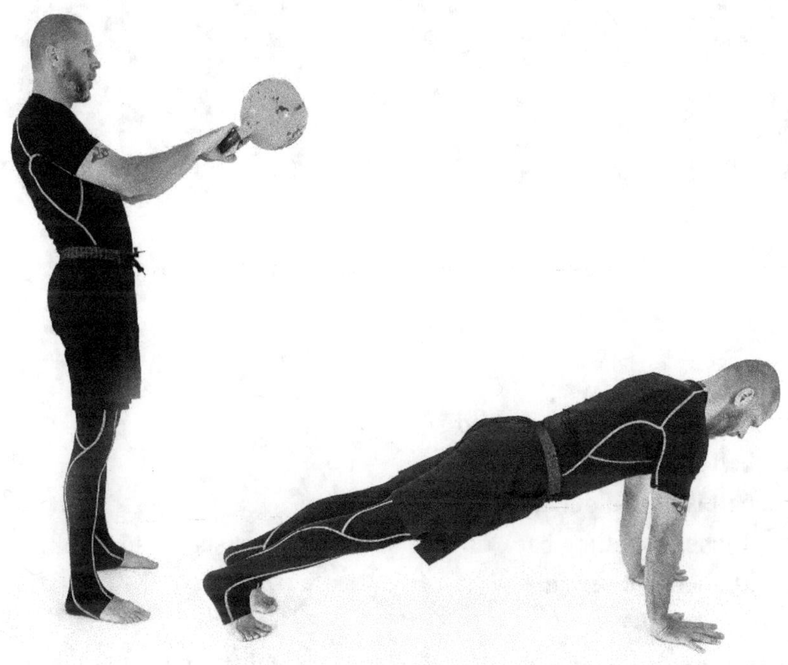

Kettlebell Swing Step-By-Step in Pictures

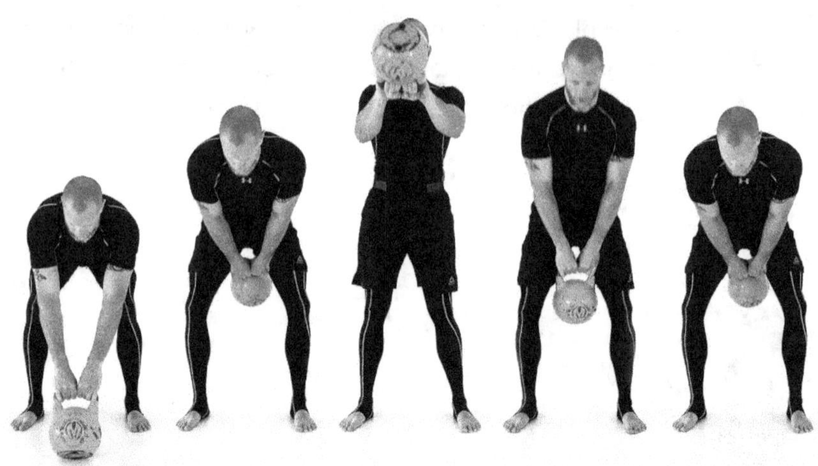

Pictured above:

1) kettlebell is dead on the ground
2) kettlebell is pulled back
3) kettlebell is pulled out and propelled forward
4) the kettlebell is falling back down and the hips just started to break
5) the kettlebell is inserted

This is the process for starting the kettlebell swing dead from the ground, if flexibility is lacking then it's perfectly okay to start the first part of the movement with a squat (see photo further down).

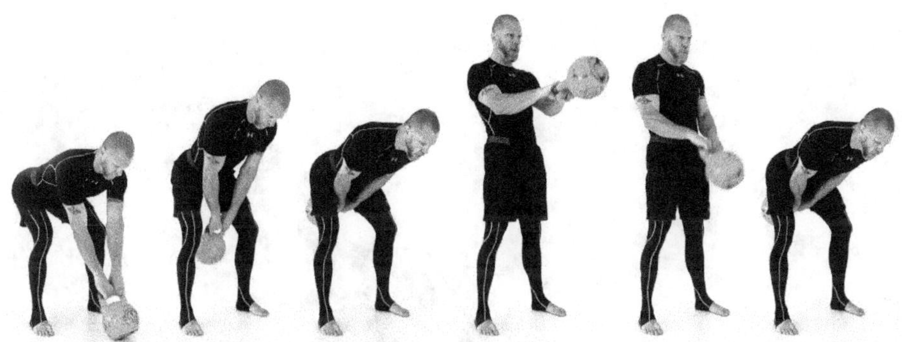

The same sequence demonstrated at a 45-degree angle.

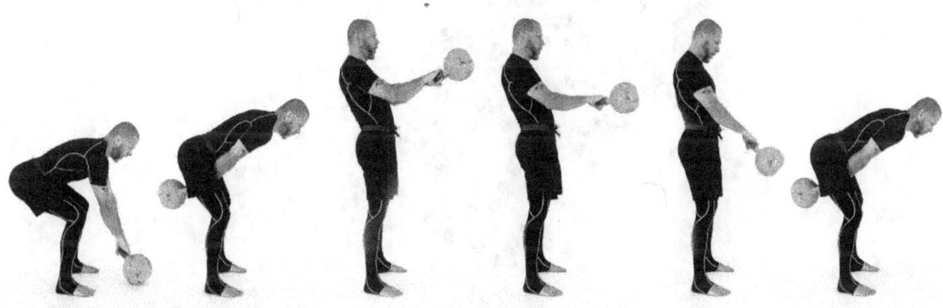

The same sequence demonstrated side-on.

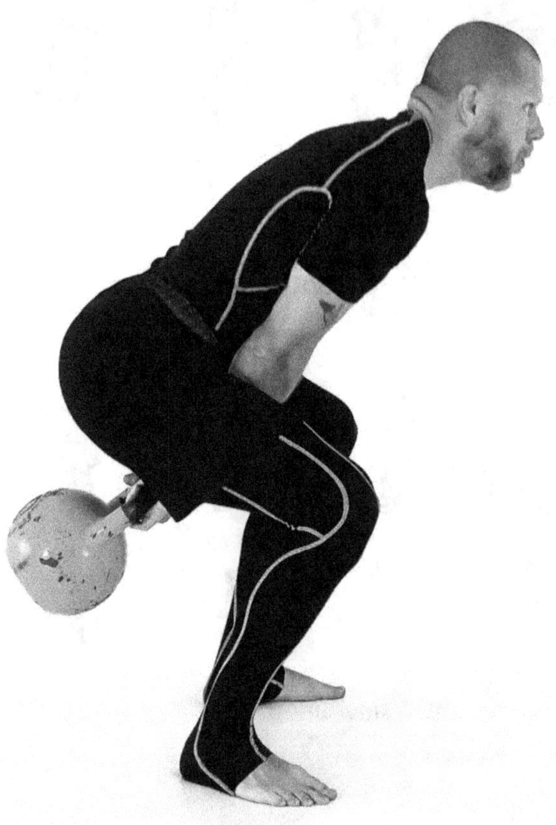

A squat movement, which can be used in the first part for pulling the kettlebell from dead into the first backswing.

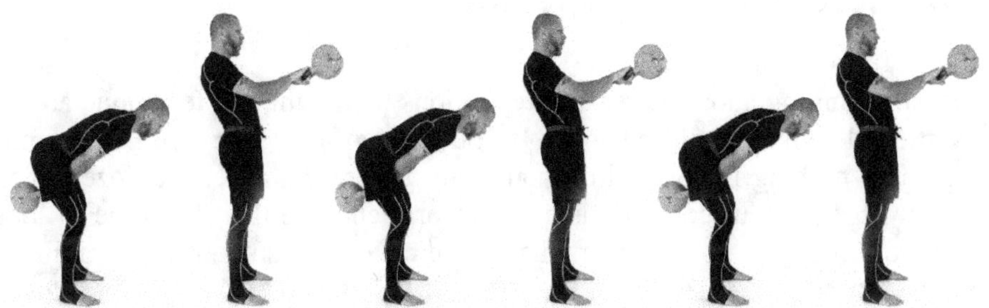

After the swing is started the above pattern is repeated.

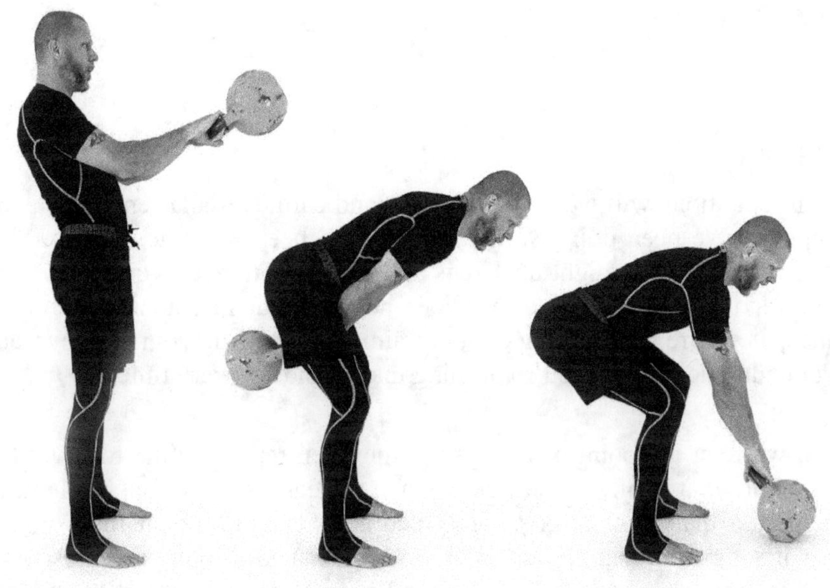

After finishing the swings the kettlebell can safely be returned back to dead the same way it was started but in reverse.

Breathing

There are several breathing patterns you can implement but the two common ones are inhale through the nose on the way down and exhale through the mouth on the way up, or exhale through the mouth when up and exhale through the mouth when down, the inhale happens automatically.

Step 4: Increasing Reps/Weight

Before even dreaming about increasing repetitions or weight, the technique and form of the kettlebell swing should be solid. If you are confident that you understand the movement and nothing is obstructing you from performing at least a dozen of solid kettlebell swings without compromising form or technique then it's time to look at how to up your training. Some factors that will dictate the results of your training, but not limited to, are:

- Unbroken repetitions
- Rest
- Volume
- Weight
- Diet

Endurance

Unbroken repetitions will work on muscular and cardiovascular endurance. Whereas everything you've been doing so far should have been with the focus on form and technique, meaning you might do 4 reps and rest for 1 minute, you might do 6, 8, or 10, whatever it is, it is a figure that does not tax your muscular or cardiovascular endurance, as you're not working out but training. Increasing your cardiovascular and muscular endurance means you're pushing that boundary every time.

Now that we're at the point of increasing unbroken reps it's time to cover the main point of failure that is often overlooked when increasing repetitions, weight, or work frequency, and that point is grip. Most people only think about the prime movers although it's the muscles responsible for grip that are doing the most work and therefore an important area to focus on and pay attention to avoid overtraining and implement a progressional increase through proper programming that aims to avoid tendonitis.

Proper progression involves listening to the body, knowing where you're at, progressively increasing what you're doing, and getting the right amount of rest to avoid overtraining and allow for proper recovery. Understanding when you've pushed too far and allowing for increased rest to recover and then continue with progression through regression.

Video of 100 unbroken kettlebell swings with medium weight: go.cavemantraining.com/youtube-100-unbroken-swings

Power

The speed and effort at which the kettlebell is swung can be changed and will affect the results of the workout at hand. The kettlebell can be pulled out and propelled away to then just let gravity take control and simply guide the trajectory in the right path, this will only provide resistance on the upswing. To get the best cardio effect from swinging the kettlebell it should be pulled out and actively inserted, resistance on both up and down for a total of approx. 80%. To go one step further and really get the most out of the kettlebell swing for the anaerobic effect (assuming the weight is heavy enough) the swing could be turned into a power swing which involves actively pulling the kettlebell down as well, 100%, i.e. there is not one moment where the kettlebell is taking advantage of gravity. The later really falls into kettlebell swing variations.

Video of 70lbs kettlebell swings: go.cavemantraining.com/youtube-70lbs-swing

Strength

Power is a combination of speed and strength, so, as you perform heavy swings know that you are not only working speed but also strength. Power training will be working in much lower rep ranging, low enough with enough rest in between sets to recover and be able to remain explosive.

Video of 105lbs swings: go.cavemantraining.com/youtube-105lbs-swing

Volume

An increase in volume is not the same as an increase in unbroken repetitions, for example, the volume of 2 sets of 100 unbroken swings is lower than 10 sets of 30 swings. Move to a higher volume over time to increase the results of cutting body fat and building muscle.

How many swings should you do?

You should do the number of swings that keep you from injury but push you in areas that your training in, i.e. the goals you're aiming to reach. The best tool to measure is your brain listening to your body, getting in tune with the effects of training, recovery, level of increase, etc. The first thing to do is decide on your goals, then understand what type of training you need to do, increase of unbroken reps, increase of weight, increase of volume, or stick with intervals, etc. Then set a starting point, a number of reps with a certain weight, record sets and rest time in between sets, record recovery between workouts, record the response of your body, and work on progression over time through adjusting your program. Don't be afraid to regress, mixing it up, rest longer, take some time off, etc.

Step 5: Working out with Kettlebell Swings

Now that you've got a good understanding of the kettlebell swings it is time to work out with the kettlebell swing and incorporate it in your workouts or build a plan around the swing itself. The following are some workouts you can work with.

Make sure you check out the muscle priming and warm-up further in this book and always make sure to warm up properly before your workout. If you want some simple ideas for warming up then stick to 10 bodyweight hip hinges, 10 jumping jacks, repeat for 4 to 6 minutes.

CTSWING1

Kettlebell Swing 12 Minute EMOM
30 kettlebell swings every minute on the minute for 12 minutes.

Perform 30 swings at the start of every minute and complete them as fast as possible, the faster you complete them the longer you have to rest, i.e. the remainder of the minute.

If you have different weights of kettlebells then you can make this more interesting by starting with your heaviest kettlebell for the first 4 minutes, then medium weight for the next 4 minutes, and finally with a lighter kettlebell for the last 4 minutes.

For my level, the following would work and you can adjust to suit yours.
- 20 x 32kg kettlebell swings for each minute of the first 4 minutes.
- 25 x 28kg kettlebell swings for each minute of the second 4 minutes.
- 30 x 24kg kettlebell swings for each minute of the last 4 minutes.

This is a workout you can do <u>approximately</u> 3 times a week. I say approximately as there are so many variables involved that it's not possible to give an accurate number for every individual.

CTSWING2
8 Minute Kettlebell Swing Intervals

The first 8 sets are 15 seconds of work and 15 seconds of rest with a kettlebell of a heavier weight you can get about 7 to 8 fast and powerful swings in.

The second 8 sets are 20 seconds of work and 10 seconds of rest with a kettlebell of a weight you can moderately easy get 10 to 12 or more power swings in.

This is a workout you can do <u>approximately</u> 5 or more times a week.

CTSWING3

20 Minute AMRAP Kettlebell Swing

Perform as many rounds as possible of the following exercises within the given time.

- 10 kettlebell swings with a moderately heavy weight or 15 with a lighter weight
- 5 bodyweight squats
- 10 jumping jacks

This is a workout you can do <u>approximately</u> 5 or more times a week.

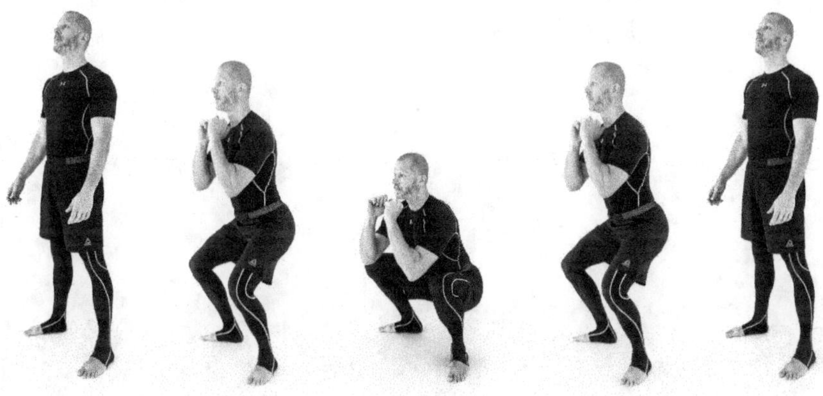

Bodyweight squats

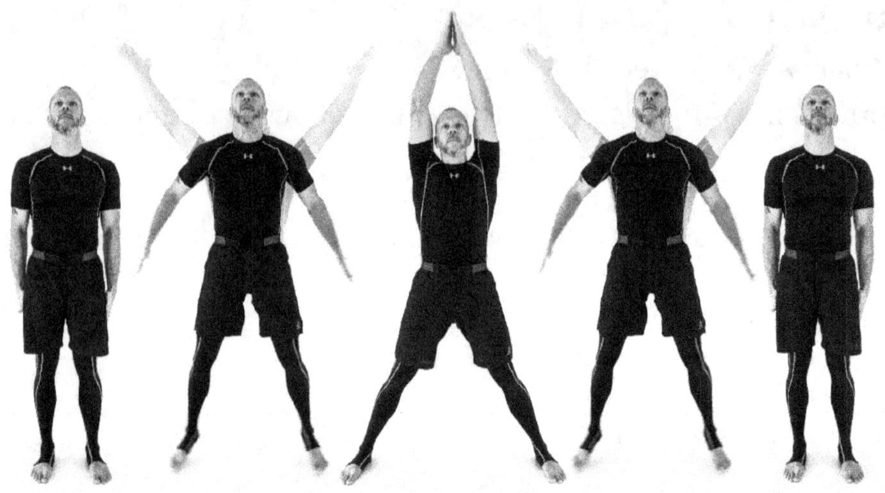

Jumping Jacks

CTSWING4

20 Minute AMRAP Kettlebell Swing

Perform as many reps as possible of the following exercises within the given time for each task.

Task 1: 4 minutes of kettlebell swings and rest for 1 minute
Task 2: 4 minutes of jumping jacks and rest for 1 minute
Task 3: 4 minutes of bodyweight squats and rest for 1 minute
Task 3: 5 minutes of kettlebell swings

Record your total number of reps and increase them over time, once you see no increase in reps then you increase weight.

This is a workout you can do <u>approximately</u> 2 or more times a week.

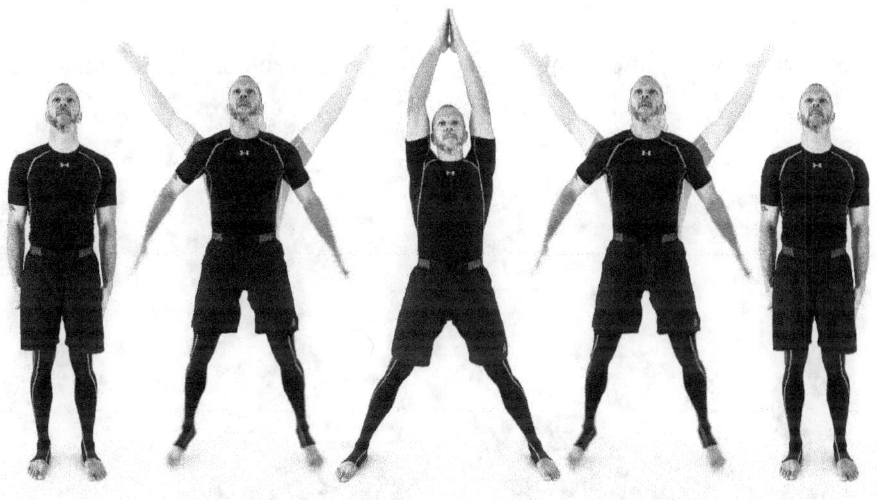

Jumping Jacks

CTSWING5

Kettlebell Swings And Burpees FOR TIME

Complete a set-out number reps of swings and burpees for the fastest time possible.

100 kettlebell swings
25 burpees
75 kettlebell swings
25 burpees
50 kettlebell swings
25 burpees
25 kettlebell swings

Record your time and try and improve it every time you repeat the workout. Use a medium-weight kettlebell. The burpees are without push-up or jump.

This is a workout you can do <u>approximately</u> 1 time a week or pull out once a month to test.

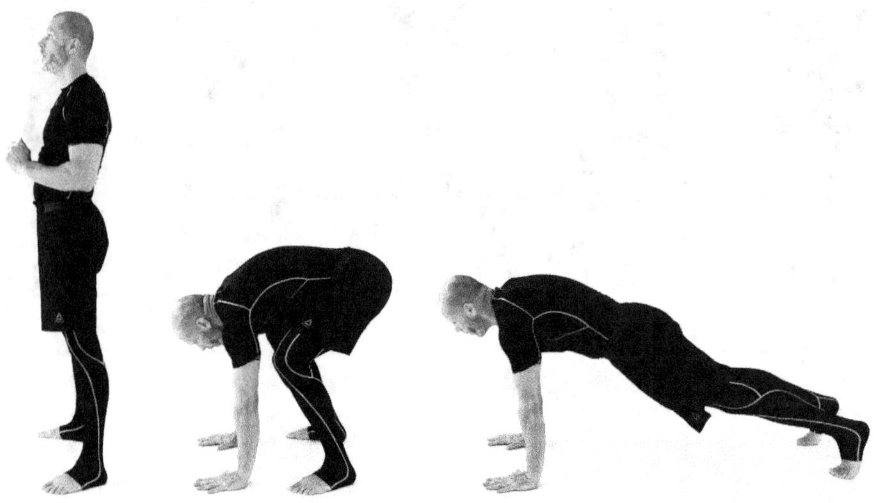

Burpee down

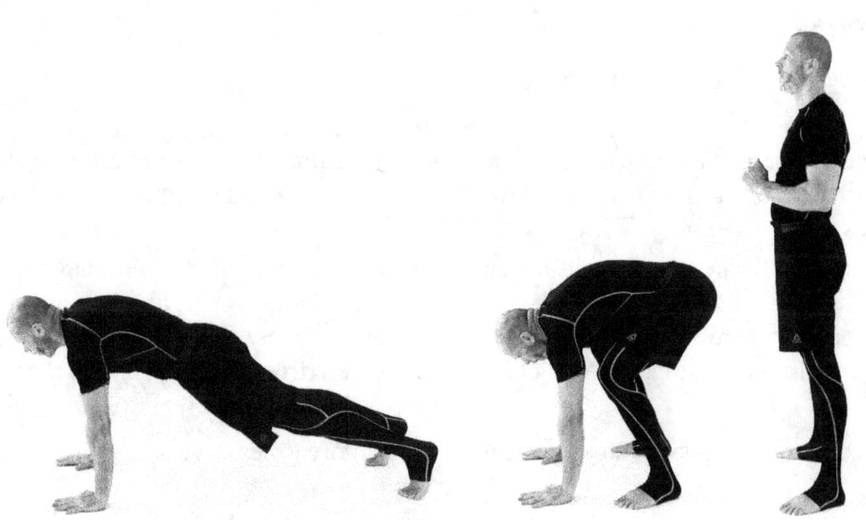

Burpee up

CTSWING6

Kettlebell Swings For Strength

Grab your heaviest kettlebell and swing it 4, 6, or 8 times and then rest for as long as is required to bring the heart rate down to normal. Repeat this sequence for 45 to 60 minutes.

The number of reps you do will depend on how heavy a kettlebell you have, for my level it would be 4 at 48kg / 105lbs, 6 at 40kg, or 8 at 36kg. The amount of rest would be anywhere from 2 minutes and up. I would use my rest time for mobility and stretching. In the session, I would complete anywhere from 16 to 20 sets or more.

This is a workout you can do <u>approximately</u> 2 or more times a week.

CTSWING7

Kettlebell Swings For Endurance

Grab a light kettlebell and warm up with 10 x 10 reps.

Grab a slightly heavier kettlebell and perform as many unbroken reps as possible. Rest for 5 to 10 minutes. Grab a heavier kettlebell and perform as many unbroken reps as possible. Make sure to stretch the forearms.

This is a workout you can do <u>approximately</u> 4 or more times a week, it will depend on how many you're able to do unbroken and what weight you're at. Remember, listen to the body.

These are just some ideas you can use to train with the kettlebell swing, join our online kettlebell community to post your results, no matter what the results are, it's only going to get better from the first time you post.

Join us here http://bit.ly/kettlebellgroup or if you prefer something more specific then join us here www.facebook.com/groups/kettlebell.swing/

COMMIT
PERSIST
CELEBRATE

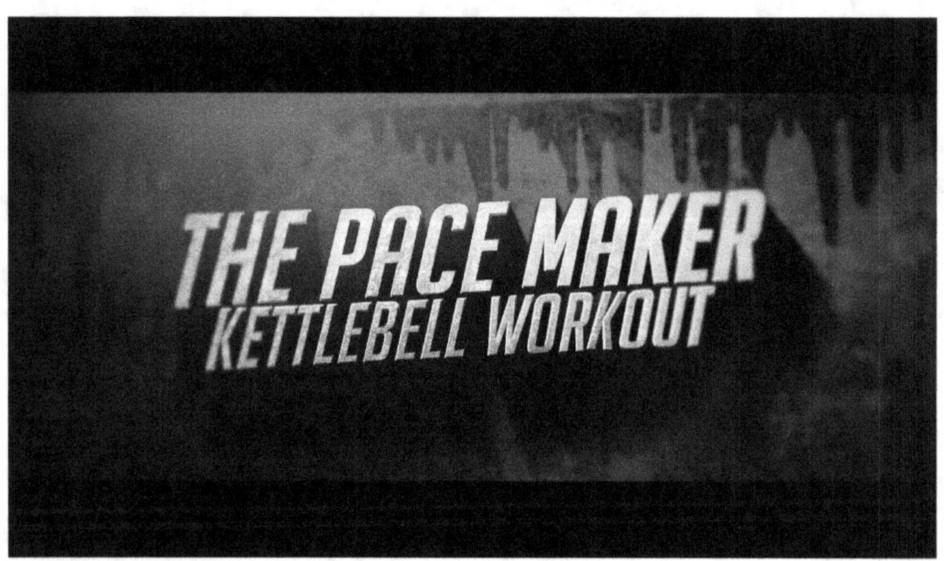

If you're ready to kick it up a notch and really seriously test not only your technique, but also mental toughness, and pacing, then have a crack at THE PACE MAKER.

The workout is simple… but insane. 1 kettlebell. Just 20 minutes. 3 Exercises.

Can you complete it? Can you complete it unbroken?

30 seconds single arm swings on one side

30 seconds single arm swings on the other side

30 seconds full snatch on one side

30 seconds full snatch on the other side

30 seconds overhead reverse lunge on one side

30 seconds overhead reverse lunge on the other side

Repeat 6 rounds

Makes a total of 18 minutes

Finish with 2 minutes of push-ups

Video: go.cavemantraining.com/pace-maker-workout

This workout includes something not covered in this book and I highly recommend you read *Snatch Physics* to learn how to snatch in 21-days or less.

Get the book: go.cavemantraining.com/snatch-physics-book

Step 6: Time to Venture Further

This guide covered the most important points of the conventional two-arm kettlebell swing, know that there is plenty more to write about just this particular exercise variation alone, but there is an enormous amount to write about when it comes to the swing and all its variations.

Some of the variations but not limited to are:

- **Conventional Swing** AKA Russian Swing
  - Single Arm (one kettlebell)
  - Single Arm Alternating (one kettlebell)
  - Double Arm (one kettlebell)
  - Double Arm (two kettlebells)
- **Squat Swing**
  - Single Arm (one kettlebell)
  - Single Arm Alternating (one kettlebell)
  - Double Arm (one kettlebell)
  - Double Arm (two kettlebells)
- **American Swing**
  - Double Arm (one kettlebell)
- **Atlas Swing**
  - Single Arm (one kettlebell)
  - Double Arm (one kettlebell)
- **Pendulum Swing** AKA Kettlebell Sport Swing
  - Single Arm (one kettlebell)
  - Single Arm Alternating (one kettlebell)
  - Double Arm (one kettlebell)
- **Short Lever Swing**
  - Double Arm (one kettlebell)
- **Side-Step Swing**
  - Double Arm (two kettlebells)
- **Side Swing** AKA Suitcase Swing
  - Single Arm (one kettlebells)
  - Double Arm (two kettlebells)
- **Walking Swing**
  - Single Arm (one kettlebell)

- Double Arm (one kettlebell)
- Double Arm (two kettlebells)

- **Reverse Walking Swing**
  - Single Arm (one kettlebell)
  - Double Arm (one kettlebell)
  - Double Arm (two kettlebells)
- **Gorilla Swing**
  - Single Arm (one kettlebell)
  - Double Arm (one kettlebell)
  - Double Arm (two kettlebells)
- **Crescent Swing**
  - Double Arm (one kettlebell)
- **Hardstyle Swing**
  - Single Arm (one kettlebell)
  - Double Arm (one kettlebell)
  - Double Arm (two kettlebells)
- **High Swing**
  - Single Arm (one kettlebells)
  - Double Arm (one kettlebell)
  - Double Arm (two kettlebells)
- **High Pull Swing**
  - Single Arm (one kettlebells)
  - Double Arm (two kettlebells)
- **Power Swing**
  - Double Arm (one kettlebell)
- And more…

For a complete list of all kettlebell exercises with videos and explanations please visit go.cavemantraining.com/**kettlebell-exercise-list** or check out the *Kettlebell Exercise Encyclopedia* by Cavemantraining™ at go.cavemantraining.com/**encyclopedia**.

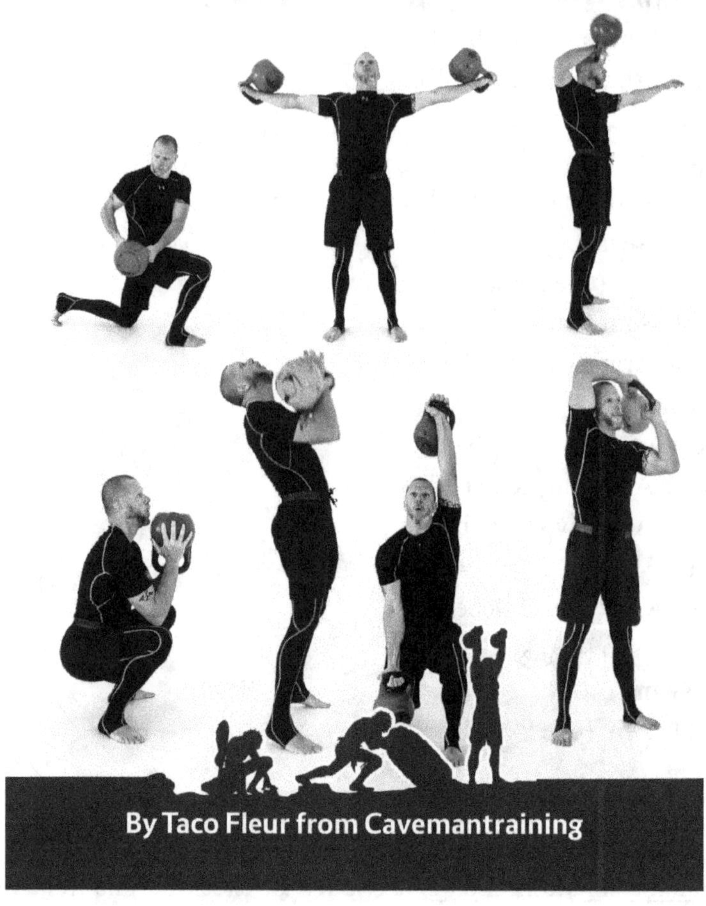

Also available as 5 volumes on Amazon.com at
go.cavemantraining.com/encyclopedia-amazon

Bonus

Please note that everything from here down is added as a bonus.

I'll start with some videos, some are not of great quality but the content is, it's a bonus that might provide additional information that not's covered in this quick guide, so, definitely worth checking out.

1) How to kettlebell swing video

go.cavemantraining.com/youtube-how-to-kettlebell-swing

2) How to swing a kettlebell correctly?

This video demonstrates different variations and covers different goals, because, to know if you're swinging correctly, you need to know what goals you're working toward.

go.cavemantraining.com/youtube-different-swings

3) Don't follow the kettlebell—Stiff lower back from kettlebell swings?

Bad quality audio but the content on following the kettlebell is great and well worth watching if you're experiencing a stiff lower back.

go.cavemantraining.com/youtube-prevent-stiff-back

4) Squat vs Hip Hinge Kettlebell Swing Side-by-side Comparison

This video does a great job clearly showing the difference in slow-motion between a swing performed with a hip hinge or a squat.

go.cavemantraining.com/youtube-hh-vs-squat

Subscribe if you want to be notified about new videos on our YouTube channel
go.cavemantraining.com/youtube-subscribe

Personalized Online Coaching

Anyone that purchased a copy of this guide can receive personalized online coaching from me, check the following link for full details on how it works and how you can take your kettlebell swing to the next level go.cavemantraining.com/**online-swing-coaching**.

What Muscles Are Worked with the Kettlebell Swing?

For those interested, the following delves deeper into the muscles used during the kettlebell swing.

The kettlebell swing is a full-body exercise that uses muscles for grip, posture, stabilization, to keep the spine erect, and the actual movement (prime movers). I cover the two-handed swing, the single-handed swing would involve a lot more action around the mid-section.

1. Grip
2. Posture/shoulders
3. Spine
4. Prime movers
5. Overhead
6. Flexion and stabilization

Grip

The muscles used for grip are usually not mentioned or thought off, however, your swing is only as good as your grip. In fact, most of your training is only as good as your grip, if you have a weak grip then you won't be lifting heavy. If your grip has no endurance then you won't be completing high reps unbroken.

Posture/shoulders

I'm referring to the top part of your body at the top of the swing where your shoulders are nice and safely pulled down. Your chest it out, shoulders blades slightly down and pulled together.

Spine

Throughout the swing, your erector spinae muscles need to work to keep your spine erect, and there is actually a lot more going on inside as well to protect the spine and brace the abs.

Prime movers

These are the muscles that create the movement which is the hip and knee extension only when we're talking about the conventional kettlebell swing.

Flexion and stabilization

The flexion I refer to is knee flexion and the stabilization I refer to is that of keeping the knee in place above the ankle. Keeping the knee above the ankle is important when hip hinging, if the knee comes excessively forward, then the movement starts to turn into a squat. A kettlebell squat swing is not bad, it's only bad if you need to perform a hip hinge and perform a squat, or perform the squat swing incorrectly, otherwise, the squat swing is an excellent exercise. See a side by side comparison of the hip hinge versus squat swing.

Grip

1. Flexor digitorum superficialis
2. Flexor digitorum profundus
3. Flexor digit minimi brevis
4. Lumbricals

Posture/shoulders

1. Rhomboideus minor
2. Rhomboideus major
3. Lower trapezius
4. Levator scapulae
5. Latissimus dorsi

Spine

1. Iliocostalis
2. Longissimus
3. Spinalis

Prime movers

1. Gluteus maximus
2. Bicep femoris (long head)
3. Semitendinosus

4. Semimembranosus
5. Adductor magnus
6. Rectus femoris
7. Vastus lateralis
8. Vastus medialis
9. Vastus intermedius

Flexion and stabilization

1. Biceps femoris
2. Semitendinosus
3. Semimembranosus
4. Gracilis
5. Sartorius
6. Gastrocnemius
7. Soleus
8. Popliteus

Ever Wondered What Exactly Happens During a Kettlebell Swing?

What muscles do what, and why? The following are the analyses of a double arm kettlebell swing with an insert.

From backswing to up phase

Hip extension

- Gluteus Maximus pulls the top of pelvis up
- Hamstrings pull on the bottom of the pelvis

AKA hip extensors

Knee extension

Quads extend the knee

Prevent ankle flexion (Plantarflexion)

Calves pull to stop the knees from coming forward

Remain erect

Spinal erectors stop the spine from falling into flexion, and keep it erect

Protect shoulders

Latissimus dorsi pull the ball into the socket to protect the shoulders

Pull shoulders back

- Middle and lower trapezius retract and pull the shoulders back
- Rhomboids major and minor retract the scapula

Elbow extension

Triceps keep the elbow extended

Whether you need to keep the elbows extended depends on the trajectory of the kettlebell, out or up?
www.cavemantraining.com/caveman-kettlebells/extended-flexed-arms-kettlebell-swing/

Finger flexion

Muscles in the anterior compartment of the forearm keep the fingers flexed to maintain a hold on the kettlebell handle

A tight grip that does not relax at the top of the swing will create tight forearms or injury with high and repetitive volume.

From floating phase to backswing

Hip flexion

The hip flexors pull the pelvis down

Hip flexors: Psoas major, Iliacus muscle, Rectus femoris, Sartorius, Tensor fasciae latae, Pectineus, Adductor longus, Adductor brevis, Gracilis.

Knee flexion

The hamstrings, gracilis, sartorius, gastrocnemius, and popliteus flex the knee joint

Insert

The knee and hip flexors pull the hips further back and down to create an insert

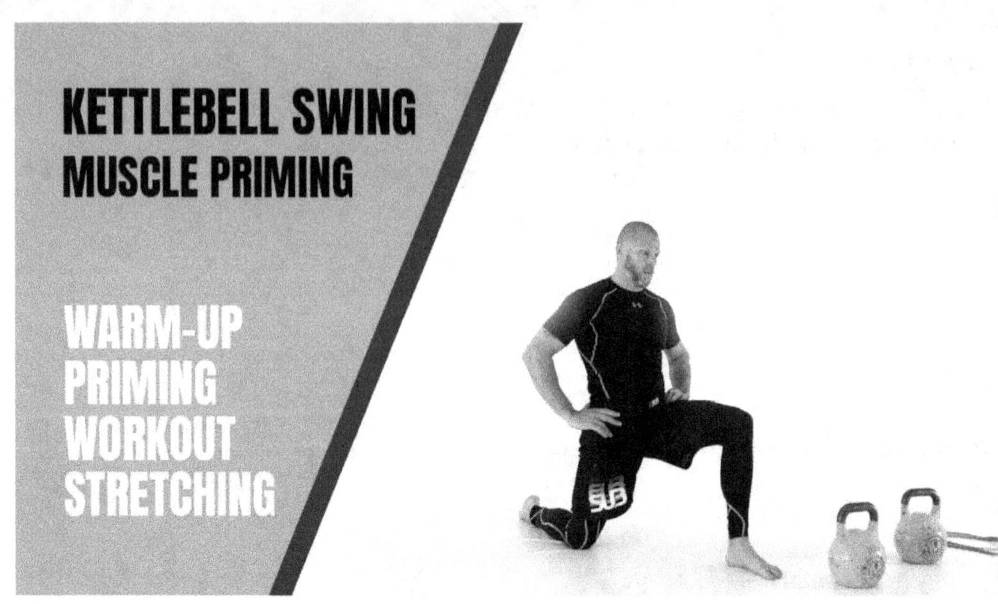

Caveman Kettlebell Swing Muscle Priming Routine

Whether you're new to the kettlebell swing or a seasoned athlete, a good routine for warming up and priming the muscles is gold. This is it.

Video go.cavemantraining.com/youtube-muscle-priming

Warm-up

The first part of the warm-up is simple and focuses on getting the hips going and warming up the body.

- 5 single leg hip circles (each side)
- 10 jumping jacks

Repeat 6 times
Approx. 3 minutes

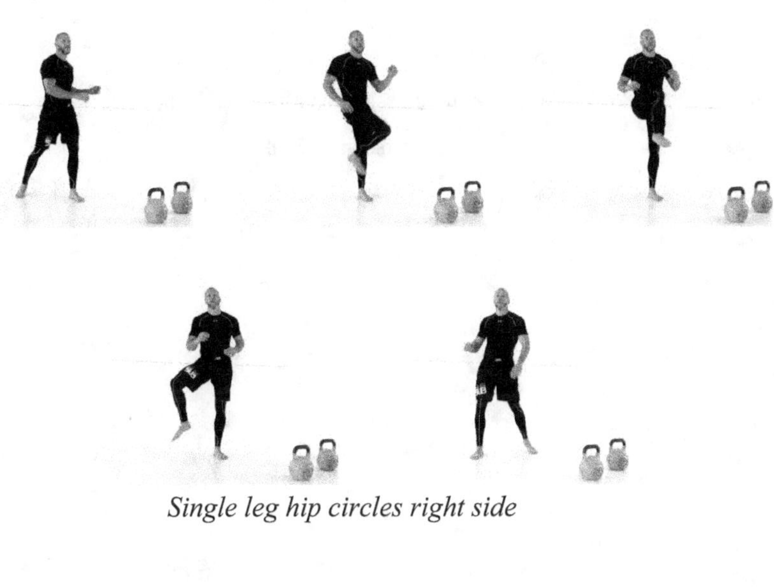

Single leg hip circles right side

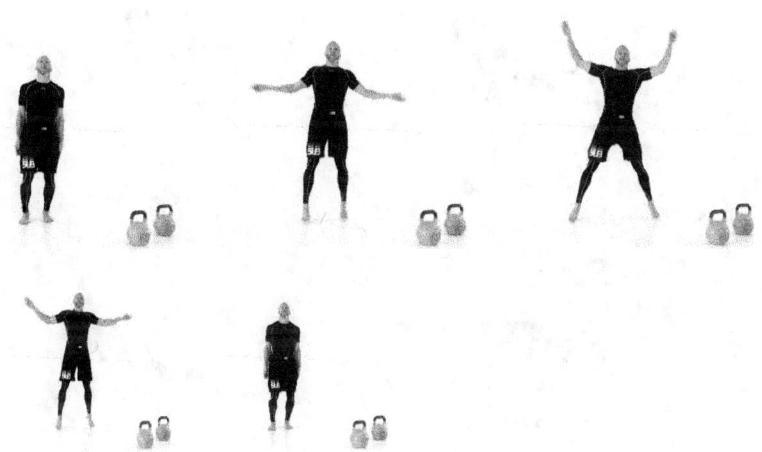

The second part of the warm-up focusses on the hips plus the posterior chain.

- Prone hip and thoracic hyperextension into pike
- Runners lunge (each side)
- Stand up

Repeat 6 times

Approx. 1 ½ minutes

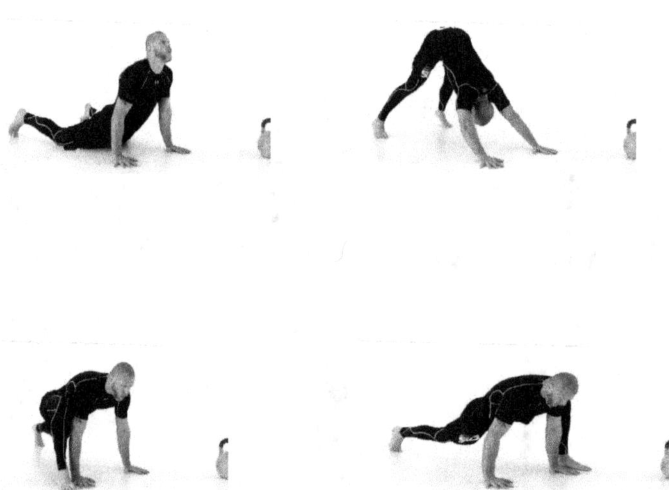

- Prone hip and thoracic hyperextension into pike
- Runners lunge and twist (each side)
- Stand up into arms overhead

Repeat 6 times

Approx. 2 minutes

Repeat the warm-up twice.

Approx. 10 minutes

Warning

Hip and thoracic hyperextension should be approached like anything, with progression and care. These two areas are usually not conditioned with the average person, this does not mean it's an area that should not be worked, it means it should be worked and progressed safely. Before you attempt this make sure you understand how to protect your lumbar and create range with the hips and thoracic.

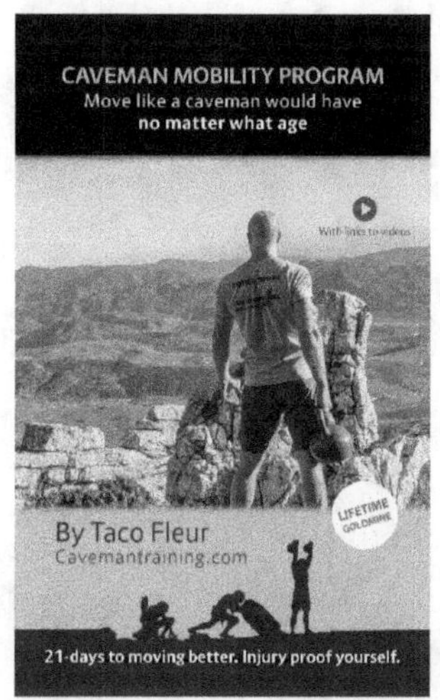

If in doubt, join our free Facebook groups and ask, or buy the book on Amazon or Cavemantraining.

Muscle priming

This is the part where you're connecting with the areas that are going to do the work for you.

The sequence is as follows:

- 5 x prone single-leg hip hyperextensions (each side)
- 5 x prone thoracic hyperextensions
- 5 x kneeling hip extensions
- Kneeling lunge 10 x pulse (each side)
- 5 x true hip hinge
- 5 x quarter squat

Repeat twice
Approx. 4 minutes

Follow up with some shoulder circles to get the upper body loose.

1) Single leg hip hyperextensions

These are to connect with the gluteus maximus and feel the area that is going to do the primary work for you during swings.

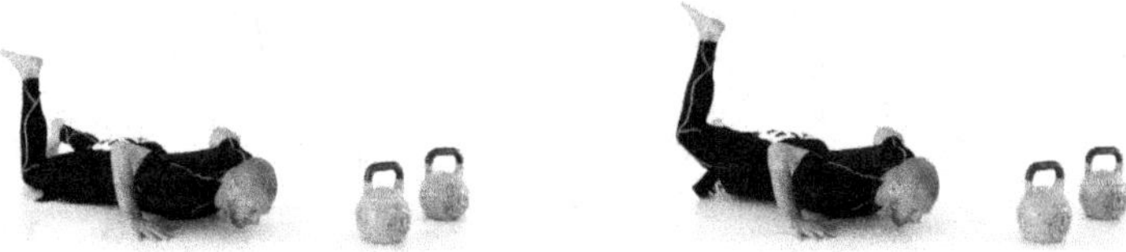

2) Prone thoracic hyperextensions

These are to connect with your erector spinae muscle groups which are to be contracted and simply hold the spine straight (erect) to be moved by the pelvis.

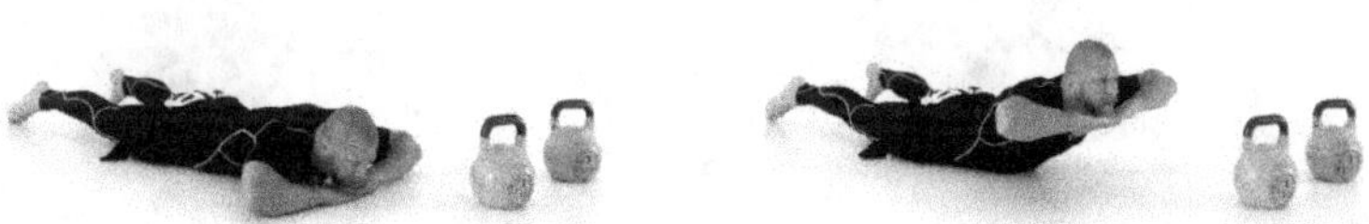

3) Kneeling hip extensions

These are to connect with hamstring muscles which will be pulling at the bottom of your pelvis and help to pull it up during the upswing.

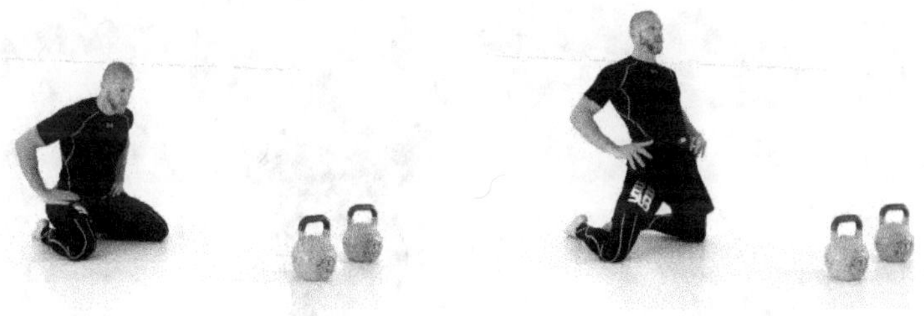

4) Kneeling lunge and pulse

The goal of these is two-fold, the pull with the front leg activates the hamstrings, and the hips coming forward digs into the psoas on the side that the leg is kneeling.

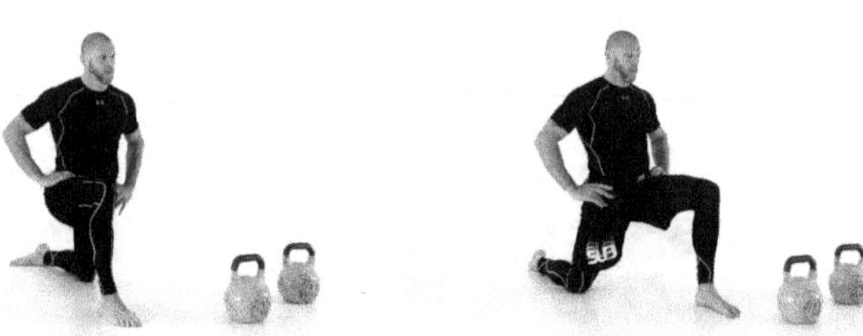

5) True hip hinge

The true hip hinge (AKA stiff-legged hip hinge) prepares you for the primal movement of the kettlebell swing.

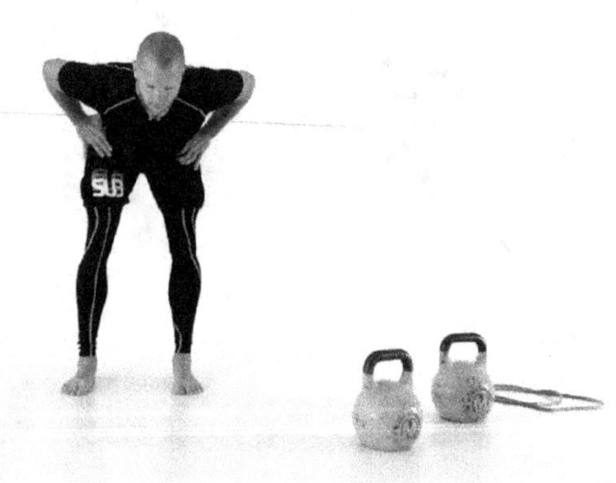

6) Quarter squat

These are to target the quadriceps which are responsible for knee extension which happens at the same time as a hip extension.

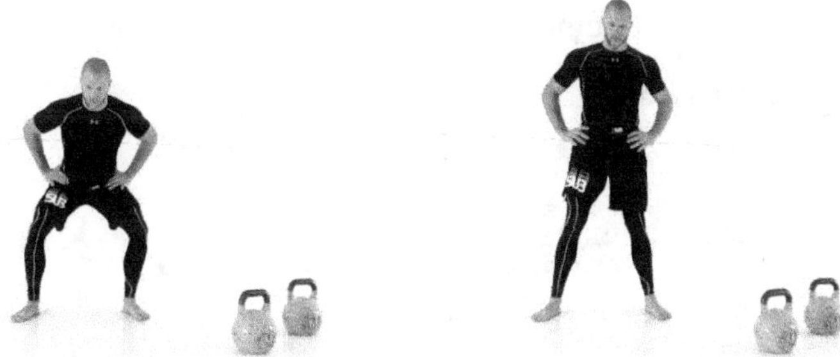

Want to learn a new workout each week?

Join the *Caveman Inner Circle* where a select group of people from across the world complete one of the Cavemantraining workouts together. Not only do you get access to a unique workout each week, access to two kettlebell coaches, and each workout has a progression or alternative, meaning anyone can do them.

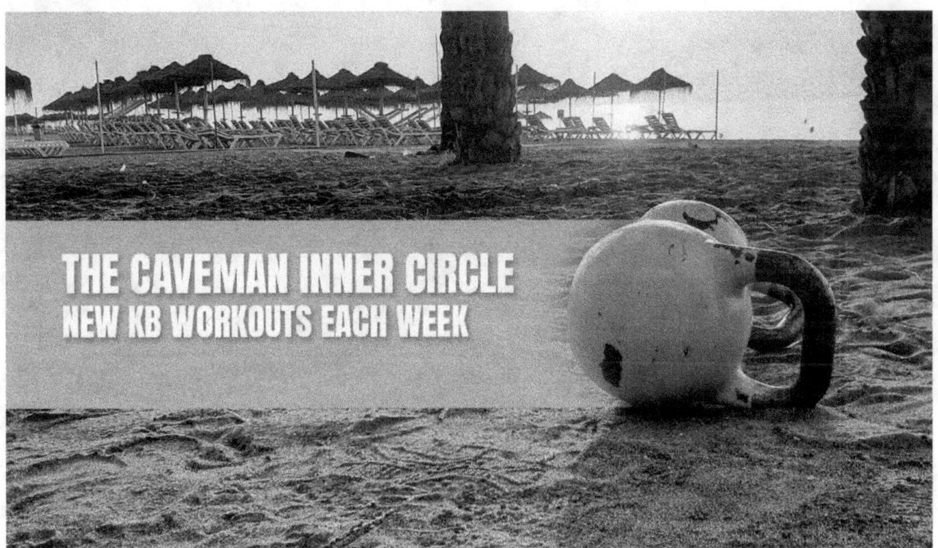

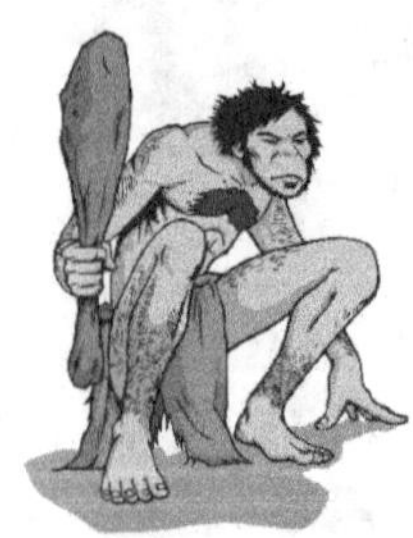

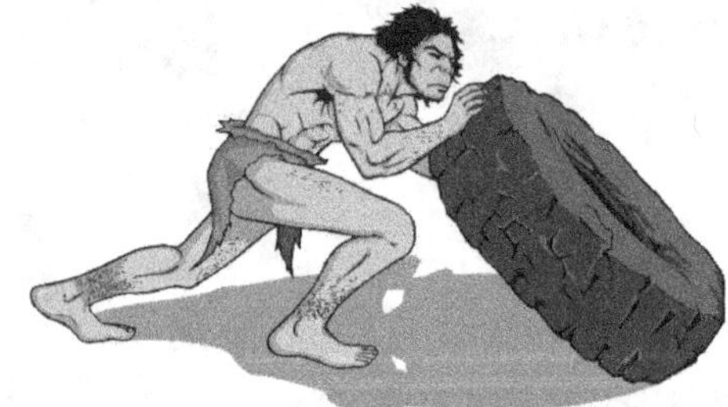

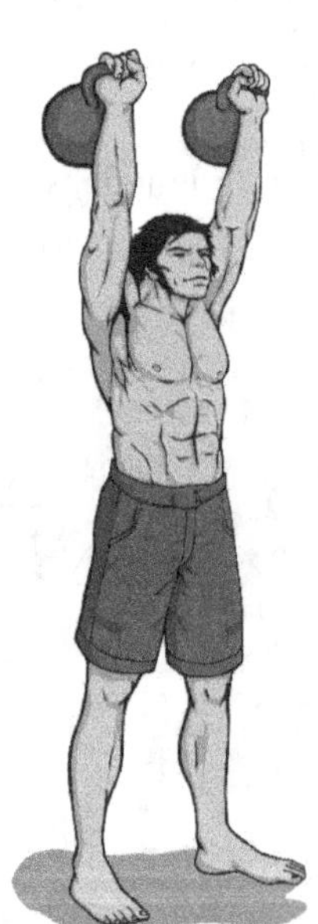

Kettlebell Books

Check out some of our other popular kettlebell books and courses:

1. 21-Days to Kettlebell Training for Beginners
2. Kettlebell Workouts and Challenges 1.0
3. Kettlebell Workouts and Challenges 2.0
4. Kettlebell Exercise Encyclopedia
5. And more

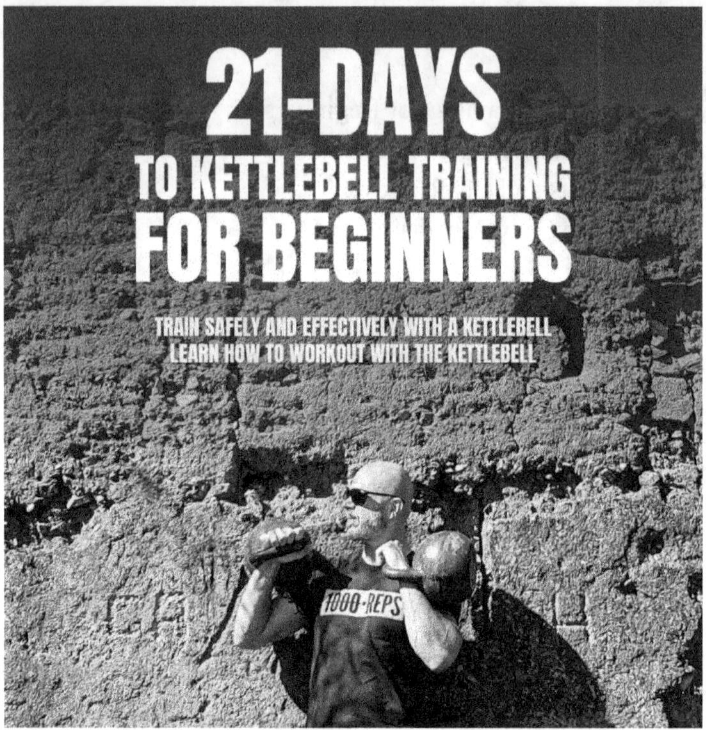

1. For the Android as a video course go.cavemantraining.com/android-video-course
2. For the computer as an online course go.cavemantraining.com/21-day-kb-course
3. DVD or Bluray go.cavemantraining.com/21-day-dvd-bluray
4. Streaming go.cavemantraining.com/21-day-streaming
5. Udemy go.cavemantraining.com/21-day-udemy coupon code: HXXPPQKT

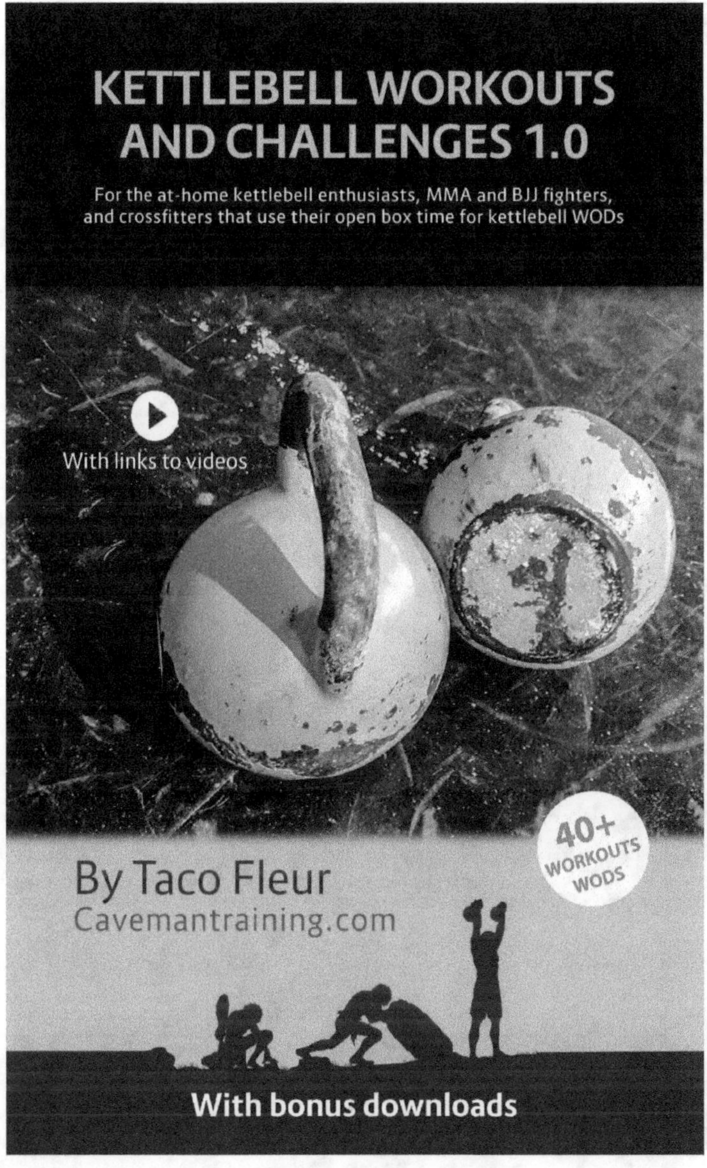

Available for direct download on Cavemantraining.com at
go.cavemantraining.com/workouts-1 or as Kindle or Paperback on Amazon.com.

Paperback: go.cavemantraining.com/workout-1-paperback
Kindle: go.cavemantraining.com/workout-1-kindle

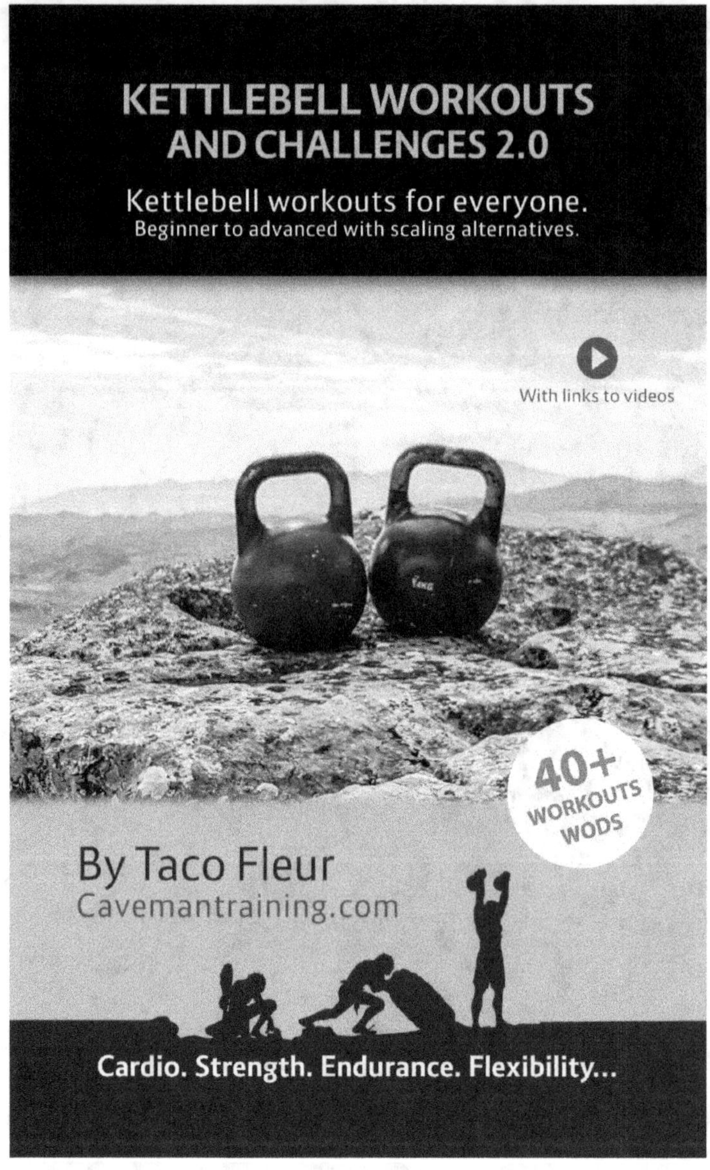

Available for direct download on Cavemantraining.com at go.cavemantraining.com/workout-2 or as Kindle or Paperback on Amazon.com.

Paperback: go.cavemantraining.com/workout-2-paperback
Kindle: go.cavemantraining.com/workout-2-kindle

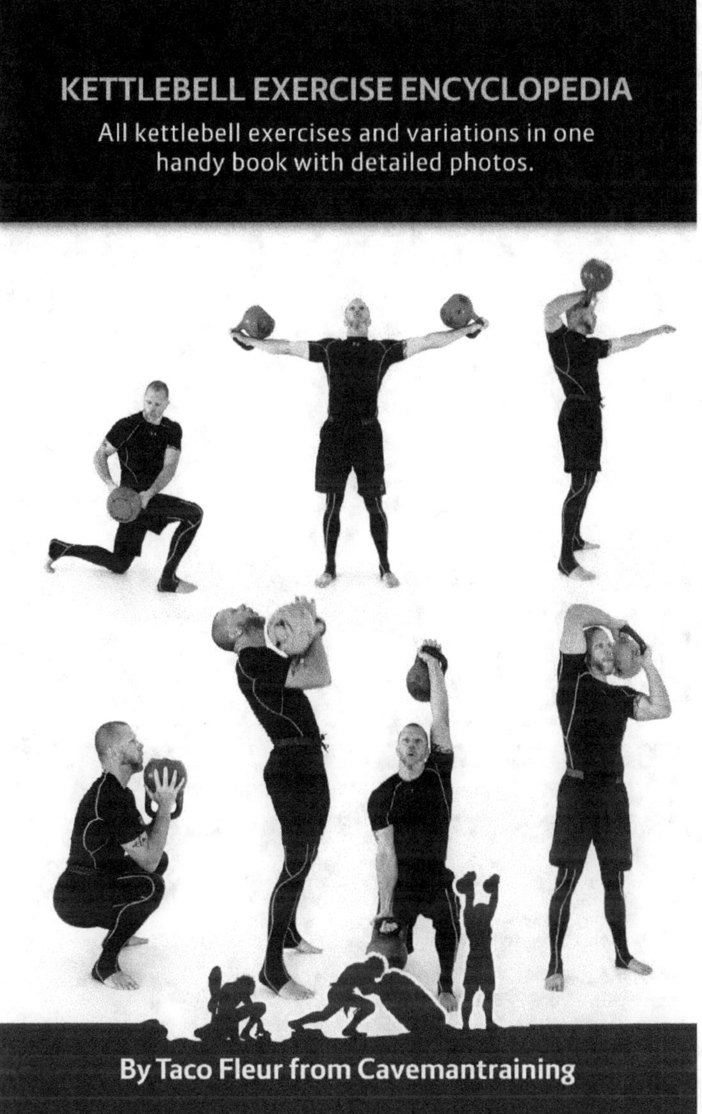

Available for direct download as one book on Cavemantraining.com at go.cavemantraining.com/encyclopedia or as 5 volumes in Kindle or Paperback on Amazon.com.

Amazon: go.cavemantraining.com/encyclopedia-amazon

Become Certified

Become certified or just complete the course to know that you are doing things right. www.cavemantraining.com/learn-kettlebells-home or check out our other online certifications here www.cavemantraining.com/online-kettlebell-courses-and-certifications

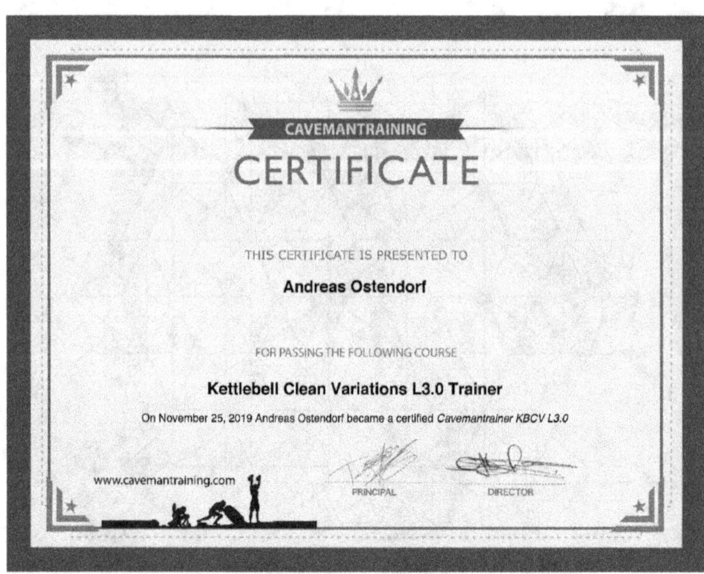

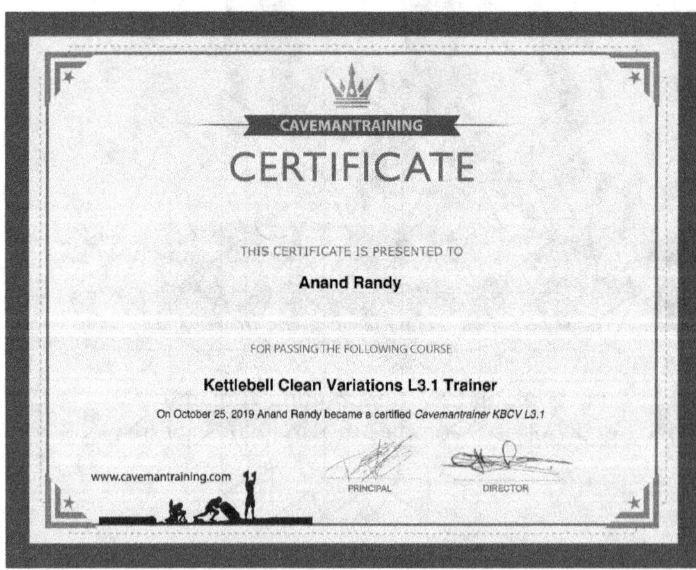

Kettlebell Features And Which Kettlebell To Get? What Size And Weight?

If you're just entering the world of kettlebell training and your budget is tight then you want to make a good choice when buying your first kettlebell(s). We've put together some extremely important information for those looking to buy a new kettlebell.

For those not wanting to get into the nitty-gritty, I will list a quick and simple opinion and for those wanting to delve deeper, I will cover all the kettlebell features.

1) If you know that you will be sticking with kettlebell training and progress one step at a time, then the competition kettlebell is for you.

2) If you're not sure about kettlebell training yet and want to test the waters or will be sticking to a few basic exercises, then a cheaper cast iron kettlebell is for you. But know that if you experience annoyances, spending a bit more money in the beginning, could have avoided that.

Whether you choose 1 or 2, make sure to avoid the Kettlebell Avoidances listed further down.

Kettlebell Features

The following describes the features of a kettlebell and how they could affect your training.

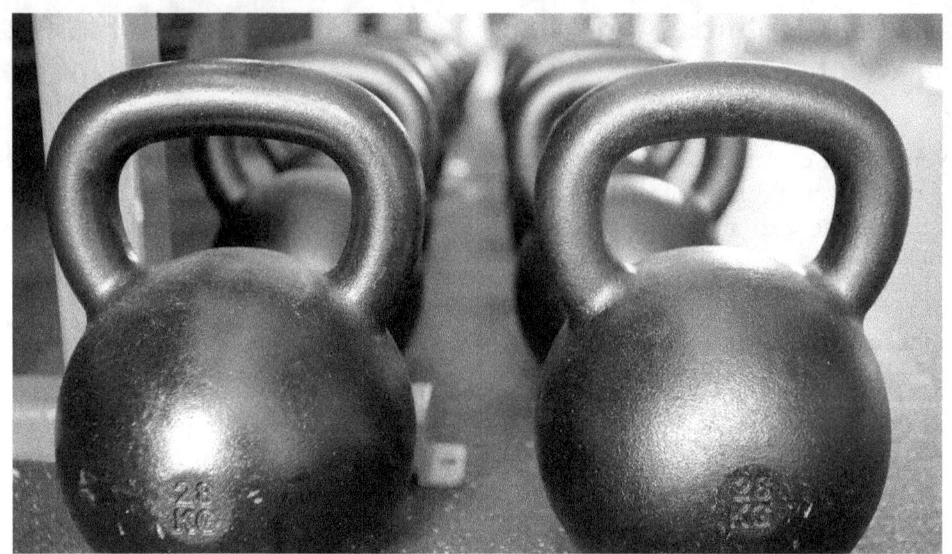

Kettlebell Handle And Window Size

Let's talk about kettlebell handle sizes and the window, in particular, the differences and why they are different. The major differences in handle/window sizes are found with cast iron kettlebells and not with competition kettlebells, as all good competition kettlebells regardless of weight should have the exact same dimensions with only the thickness of the handle changing between the standard 33mm and 35mm.

The bell of a competition kettlebell remains the size whether you get an 8kg or 48kg, whereas cast iron kettlebell increase in size as the weight goes up. That increase applies to the bell and the handle. More about that further down.

Competition Kettlebell vs Cast Iron

At Cavemantraining we promote and prefer competition kettlebells for many reasons, but we also believe in being able to work with both. The competition kettlebell doesn't require changes in regards to racking or other positions when it comes to an increase in weight, whereas the cast iron bells do require changes and adjustments.

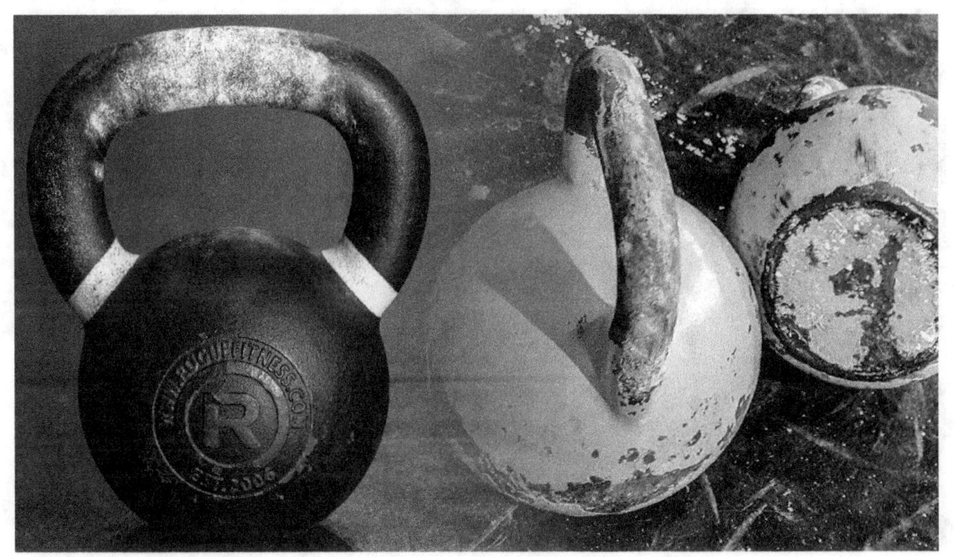

Competition Kettlebell	Cast Iron Kettlebell
Steel	Iron
More durable	Less durable
Same size	Changes in size
Color-coded	Not always color-coded
Less grip fatigue	Increased grip fatigue
More space required for two bells	Easier to work with two bells
Bigger base	Smaller base
More suited for juggling	Not well suited for juggling
More expensive	Cheaper
Same size handle	Handle narrow or wider
Rectangle-shaped handle	V-shaped handle

Color-coded

Competition kettlebells are always color-coded whereas cast iron kettlebells are only recently starting to be color-coded with a color-coded ring around the horn(s) of the kettlebell. go.cavemantraining.com/kettlebell-color-coding

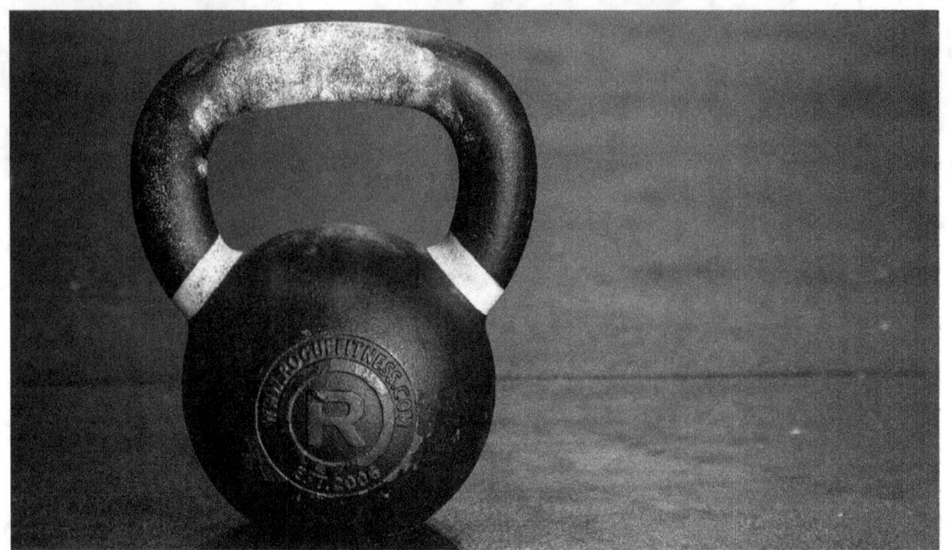

Grip fatigue

A larger diameter handle means a tighter grip for most people, which results in early grip fatigue.

Steel vs Iron

Steel is harder and stronger than cast iron, approximately 30 to 40% stronger and therefor the bigger handle diameter when the weight increases, the more reliable it will be.

Double kettlebell work

Double kettlebell work is easier for shorter people as there isn't as much space between the legs required, whereas two competition kettlebells require a lot more space. During cleans, swings, snatches, etc. this could mean having to step out to the side and in upon each rep.

Base size

The base of the competition kettlebell is larger than the base of the cast iron kettlebells which makes the competition kettlebell more suitable for exercises like push-ups, L-sits, plank, burpees, etc.

Handle width

If you have large hands and intend to do a lot of kettlebells swings with two hands then a cast iron kettlebell with a wider handle/window might be the option for you. From personal experience, I find that a wider handle is great for double hand swings but that's all it's great for, as for anything single hand, which is most exercises, the width of the handle becomes very uncomfortable.

When you are going to press extremely heavy weights overhead then a thicker handle will provide a larger surface to distribute pressure within the palm, hence, potentially making the pressure of the handle within the palm less painful.

The reason for competition kettlebell handles/windows being smaller than most cast iron kettlebells is because as the name suggests, they were designed for kettlebell competitions which only involves one-handed exercises.

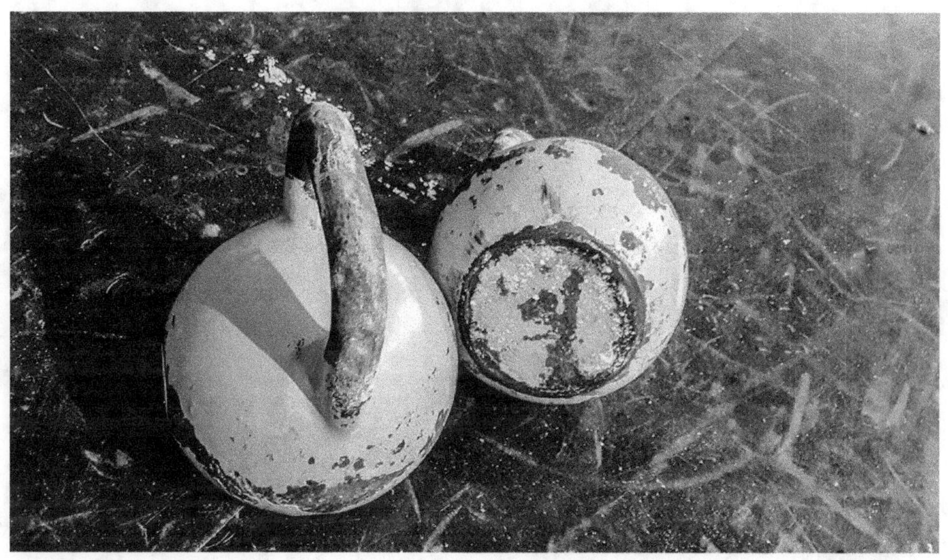

Handle shape

The shape of the handle for the competition kettlebell resembles more of a rectangle whereas the cast iron kettlebells commonly have more a V-shaped design. The v-shape design makes it easier to hold with some grips, however, the same exercises can be performed with different but just as comfortable grips with the competition kettlebell. Get a free copy of the kettlebell grip PDF to see over 25+ grips in action. go.cavemantraining.com/kettlebell-grip-pdf

ANATOMY OF THE KETTLEBELL

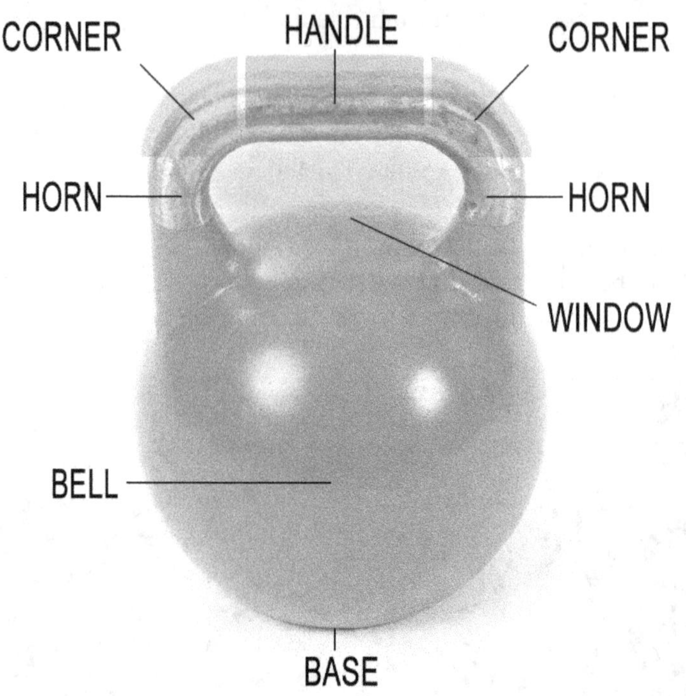

ILLUSTRATED: COMPETITION KETTLEBELL

1. Kettlebell Handle
2. Corner(s)
3. Horn(s)
4. Window
5. Bell
6. Base

Kettlebell Avoidances

In the end, try both and see which one you prefer, but make sure that whatever kettlebell you get, it does not have:

- rough spots (seams or ridges)
- loose filling
- imprints

If the kettlebell is made out of two molds as opposed to one, then it might have rough seams or ridges that can eventually become annoying and/or create blisters. If the kettlebell has fillers then this might come loose at some stage and rattle, which becomes extremely annoying. If the kettlebell has a logo or text imprinted then this can become annoying on the forearm and/or get sharp edges that will wear at clothing.

If you want to know more and in particular what kettlebell weight to choose then check out the free PDF that provides all those answers. go.cavemantraining.com/what-kettlebell-weight

Vinyl, Adjustable, KettlebellConnect, or Other Kettlebells

We do not recommend anything other than competition or iron cast kettlebells with the plain reason being, none of these other options are for serious kettlebell enthusiasts, and they're only good for a couple of exercises, and those are usually executed poorly due to the filling, grip, weight distribution, etc. Although money has been offered, we stand by our principles and only promote the best.

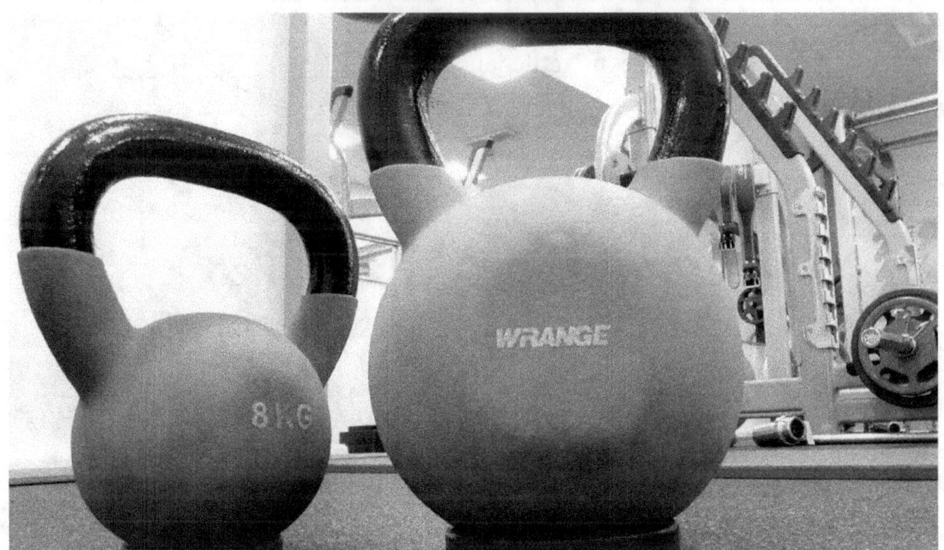

Should you get a second-hand kettlebell?

Absolutely! From a personal point of view, there is nothing better than a worn-in kettlebell, it adds character, it feels like it has more value, and there is absolutely no difference between a chipped/rusty kettlebell in regards to performance with a new one, other than you needing to sand it down a bit. I have actually paid just as much as a new kettlebell for two pairs of old and used kettlebells because they just felt good (they had soul). To me a kettlebell is more than just a piece of iron/steel, it's a piece of my life!

- Kettlebell grip PDF
  www.cavemantraining.com/shop/ebook/kettlebell-grip-ebook/
- Kettlebell starting weight PDF
  www.cavemantraining.com/caveman-kettlebells/weight-kettlebell/
- Kettlebell videos
  https://kettlebell.video/
- Kettlebells YouTube
  http://youtube.com/cavemantraining
- Kettlebell books
  www.cavemantraining.com/the-best-kettlebell-training-books/
- Kettlebell workouts
  www.cavemantraining.com/ultimate-kettlebell-workouts/
- Kettlebell courses
  www.cavemantraining.com/online-kettlebell-courses-and-certifications/
- Kettlebell DVDs
  www.cavemantraining.com/kettlebell-videos/kettlebell-dvds-for-beginners-kettlebell-training-dvds/

Become kettlebell certified

www.cavemantraining.com/online-kettlebell-courses-and-certifications/

Thank You

A big thank you from myself and the Cavemantraining team for purchasing this book, I sincerely hope that it will get you started on your amazing kettlebell journey!

I hope you'll join us in one of our many groups on Facebook to say hello.
http://bit.ly/kettlebellgroup

It's always great to hear what people think about the content, so, if you can find a few spare moments of your time and leave a review on our website, Facebook, or Amazon, that would be greatly appreciated.

It's even more appreciated if you contact us directly for any suggestions or improvements you may have.
info@cavemantraining.com or me@tacofleur.com